THE SIMPLE & HEALTHY FOOD RELATIONSHIP

A Basic Nutritional Guide for a Healthy Lifestyle... That Lasts a Lifetime

Brian Vernetti

For information contact:
Brian Vernetti
www.intervalathlete.com

Edits and formatting by Shannon Rowland. For more information, contact shannone.rowland@gmail.com.

ISBN-13: 978-1547146826
ISBN-10: 1547146826

First Edition: June 2017

To my Mother
Who always taught me to stand strong in the Truth
during times of adversity and challenge

Contents

PART TWO: Picking the Right Food

Introduction

If you are looking for a short-term diet program or quick weight loss plan, you have opened the wrong book. Understand this is not a diet book. It is, however, a nutritional guide to help you make better lifestyle decisions about the food you eat. So, if you picked up this book searching for an effective way to lose weight or gain nutritional understanding in a world full of food confusion, then you are in the right place.

But why combine two unrelated things, food and love? Because they are more related than you might expect. Forming the right bond with food is crucial to living a healthy and exciting lifestyle. Our relationship with food is something we have taken for granted as a society, and the results are drastic increases in poor heart health, shorter lifespans, and decreases in the quality of life. As a full-time Firefighter and EMT and a part-time Certified Personal Trainer, I see the direct impact of poor eating habits day-in and day-out. In order to help those around me, I knew nutrition needed to be easier to understand and also applicable for everyday situations.

Not every relationship is a good one, and that may be the case with your current eating habits. Eating healthy can be difficult at times, especially if you are unaware of what to eat. However, once you break down that barrier and become informed, your relationship with food will benefit greatly. I've designed this guide to help you succeed when confronting everything "food" out there, by informing you about nutrition, the best food choices, and practical methods, all of which will empower you to experience the many benefits of healthy eating.

You will soon possess nutritional knowledge and develop motivating factors to thrive in your food relationship.

While many other diets and weight-loss programs leave you hungry, moody, and stacking that weight back on after you are done with them, this nutritional guide will do just the opposite. You will be prepared from day one with what foods to pick, what foods to cherish, and which ones to reject. You will also get to eat the foods you love, enjoy your favorite drinks, and have great nights out on the town.

Quick References

Before jumping to the first chapter, keep an eye on the quick reference boxes below. They will guide you and point out awesome little tips to help you be victorious every day. Get ready to enjoy a great relationship with food because you deserve to be healthy and enjoy life to its fullest.

Health Awareness

Your health is #1. These boxes give helpful facts about what to look for and watch.

Remember

Important material to keep in mind.

Top Picks

My top picks for practical and tasty foods.

Food Phrase

Just a little something to help you remember important concepts.

Clear the Misconception

Not everything out there is founded on truth, but this box will guide you.

PART ONE:

Building a Foundation

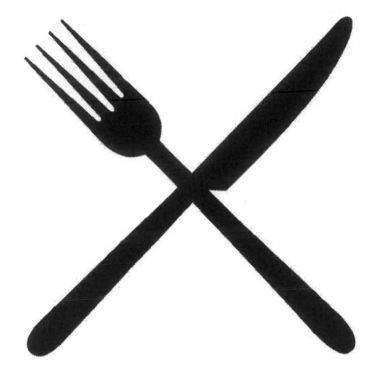

Falling Head Over Heels for Awesome Food

Intrinsic – *adjective in·trin·sic \in-'trin-zik, -'trin(t)-sik\ "Belonging to the essential nature or constitution of a thing."*

Motivation – *noun mo·ti·va·tion \ mō-tə-'vā-shən\ "A reason or reasons for acting or behaving in a particular way."*

Intrinsic Motivation – *"The driving force within us that allows us to persevere through various trials and tribulations, knowing that the results will be worth it." - Brian Vernetti*

Anytime you feel no connection or spontaneity with someone, it makes falling in love nearly impossible. The same goes for food. We need to have a unique connection with food that is practical and simple, applicable to daily life, and most importantly, healthy. So what is necessary to develop this deep connection with healthy foods? I'm glad you asked because it all starts with you.

Nutritional confusion is especially prevalent in our present society, where we are so easily overwhelmed by the myriad of false information and often led astray by fancy ad campaigns. This frustration can lead to relying on taste buds alone, which is a sure path to nutritional heartbreak. If you want to fall head over heels for awesome food, start with your internal motivation. If you have no true desire for change, then all your subsequent efforts will be futile.

You clearly already have some desire for change, which is why you're reading this book, but dig a little deeper and start asking more questions to discover what's fueling your motivation. The more questions you can answer, the stronger foundation your nutritional relationship will be.

> ➢ Do I want to lose weight? Gain weight?
> ➢ Do I want to fit into my old clothes? Get back to the weight I once was?
> ➢ Am I preparing for a wedding or event?
> ➢ Do I have concern for my health or the health of my family?
> ➢ Is my doctor recommending weight loss?

If neither the fit of your clothing nor your reflection in the mirror seem enough to motivate change, then maybe science can provide a little extra fuel to ignite that intrinsic motivation. Scientific data backing a healthy diet can be one of the most convincing arguments for the importance of eating healthy. Over the past several decades, science has proven that a healthy diet contributes to a healthy body. A healthy diet strengthens the immune system, develops stronger bones (decreases the risk of osteoporosis), increases energy levels, promotes faster healing, and even reduces early morbidity and comorbidities.

Developing a healthy food relationship decreases your risk of developing long-term health problems (comorbidities) like heart disease, diabetes, and cancer, as well as reducing the risk of stroke, high blood pressure, and high cholesterol. Eating healthy can also improve mental and emotional health, which can be a primary factor in keeping your motivation ramped up all day long. Once we understand the importance of something, it is much harder to forget or dismiss. This is especially true with nutrition. You will find that your relationship with healthy food is absolutely worth falling head over heels.

However, regardless of the reasons that you may be looking for a change, **the desire to want to change is the most important thing**. This is your intrinsic motivation. Keep this motivation in the forefront of your mind throughout this arduous journey. You will need it.

My journey began as a child. I grew up in your typical suburban home, eating typical junk food that everyone else did. I had no reason to eat anything healthy, as I simply relied on my taste buds for determining what food I would eat. I never really thought about nutrition until we experienced an unexpected family emergency.

My mother informed me that a close family member had a heart attack, requiring immediate surgery to relieve several blocked arteries and help the heart begin functioning as it normally should again. The surgery was a success, but it was a close encounter with death. The doctors ordered an immediate lifestyle change that incorporated a healthy diet and regular exercise. Little did I know, this single event would motivate me in more ways than one.

Days after the event, my mother took it upon herself to facilitate the process of eating healthy. She went through our home, throwing away all the junk food and unhealthy treats that my family and I were accustomed to devouring all day—every day. I was so dependent on unhealthy foods that I simply didn't know what to do when it came to eating right. I was confused and definitely not happy. After the initial shock receded though, I began to look at the bigger picture. Despite being only 14 at the time, I was old enough to understand that some sacrifices were necessary to improve not only my family's health but also the life of the family member who experienced the major cardiac event.

This event, along with many others that I have experienced since, has instilled a sense of self-value and motivation that I know others can experience as well. I don't want to look back on life and regret what I have done. I don't want to miss out on a life that I could have had because I ate poorly. I don't want my family to miss out on my life because of my unhealthy eating habits.

Love Connection Questions

Whether you realize it or not, you're already in a food relationship. Maybe you fell head over heels for a bad one years ago. Maybe you had a great, healthy food relationship, but before you knew it that midnight cheating with ice cream spiraled out of control into a full-on affair with junk food. Without consciously making a choice, you committed to an unhealthy relationship that's been wreaking havoc on your body and your future. It's time to discover what makes you tick and what your vices are. After all, the best way to determine what is best for you is to know yourself first.

Here are a few quick questions to help evaluate and recognize aspects of your current food relationship:

What are your motivating factors for wanting to eat healthier?

Which foods are your vices? (Chips, candy, cake, salty foods, burgers, cheese, etc.)

What do you think is the biggest hindrance to preventing you from eating healthy?

If you could change one thing about your diet, what would it be?

When was the last time you went to the doctor for a physical?

Do you know how many calories you consume every day? Rough estimate?

How many times do you eat out a week? (Fast Food, Restaurants, Take Out, etc.

What have been your struggles with food in the past?

If you were marooned on a desert island, what food could you not live without?

Hopefully these questions make you think about where you currently stand with food, what motivates you, and what has been holding you back. Keep in mind that getting to a healthy nutritional relationship is just like any other relationship— sometimes you need to break up with the junk first, figure out your type, and avoid bad influences. Knowing these things about yourself will prepare you for the next step: dating.

Getting Ready to Go on a Food Date

We have all experienced a variety of relationships. Some are good, some bad, and others, well, we don't want to even talk about those. The food in your home, the food you purchase, and those you eat regularly affect this relationship directly.

There is no doubt that when we are hungry we eat what is close and convenient, so the most important place to start improving our relationship is in our homes. The food behind the doors of your cabinets, pantries, refrigerators, and freezers are most likely the culprits of your poor eating habits. This will be the first test of your commitment.

Keep in mind that physical change begins when you start to eliminate bad temptations and embrace healthy ones. **If you don't have unhealthy foods around you, you can't indulge in them or get caught up in mindless eating.** The better foods you have, the better you will eat.

Any good relationship is founded on the things that matter most: trust, love, and time. Do you trust (know) that the foods you are eating are beneficial? Do you love how they taste? Are they able to be prepared in a timely manner?

Five Methods to Stop Dating the Wrong Food

Dating the right food is just as important as dating the right person. Although this list may seem difficult to implement at first, it is worth the sacrifice when considering the big picture of your health. Once you get rid of an unhealthy option, replace it with a healthier one. You'll soon realize that a better choice will bring you more fulfillment in the end.

Get Rid of Instant and Microwaveable Foods

Our society loves things that are quick and easy, but that doesn't mean they are good for you. Something quick n' easy, like the floozy at the bar, is a quick trip to trouble.

The only exceptions to instant and microwaveable foods are microwaveable vegetables in steamable bags.

If you have food anywhere in your kitchen that only requires a quick pop into the microwave, throw it away. Your body pays the price for convenience. Instant meals are higher in sodium, fat, and sugar—all of which are key components of an unhealthy diet. Any foods that are microwaveable most likely contain high levels of preservatives, artificial flavors, artificial colors, sodium, and sweeteners to extend their shelf lives and increase flavor—stuff you don't want or need.

Check Expiration Dates

Foods that are worth eating should expire in a relatively short time span. If you have packaged foods (chips, creams, pop tarts, jellies, gummies, condiments, meats, etc.) that last much longer than one might expect, get rid of them. Three months is a good rule of thumb for items in your cabinets and refrigerator. The longer something lasts, the more preservatives that have been added to them.

Extended shelf lives are an easy way for food companies to make more money. Food products with longer shelf lives mean less overall production and increased revenues. Just because the food companies make foods with extended shelf lives (same as instant microwaveable foods), does not mean they are healthy for you. The preservatives in food are not natural, and therefore not in our body's best interest.

A definitive time frame cannot be given for all foods as the spectrum is too broad, but *the sooner the expiration date, the better*. Toss all food that won't expire for many months to come.

Exceptions to expiration dates are those of dried beans, frozen vegetables, pastas and canned goods.

Check the Ingredients List

This concept goes hand-in-hand with expiration dates. The more ingredients that are on the back, the more likely it is chemically refined. There is a high probability that foods containing a plethora of crazy ingredients also have an extended shelf life.

The fewer ingredients in food, the better. If you haven't heard of the ingredients listed on the side, it is best to stay away from that food. Search online for each of the ingredients that are not familiar. What you will find will surprise you and change your mind next time you think of eating that food.

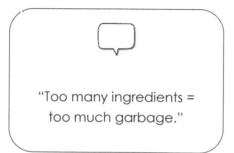

"Too many ingredients = too much garbage."

Avoid Highly Packaged or Perfectly Shaped Foods

The old saying "there ain't nothin' like the real thing" rings true with love and food.

Packaging is inevitable, but buying items that are "less" packaged is ideal. If you buy food that is subdivided into meals or packets, it is more likely to be highly processed and contain plenty of stuff you shouldn't want to eat. Also, any food that has an identical shape for each item (chicken nuggets, sweets, processed meats, tater tots, etc.) has been fed through processor after processor to create those shapes. Various ingredients

When cleaning up your food relationship, certain foods and sweets may be harder to eliminate than others.

(probably ones you have never heard, yet again) are utilized to hold those foods together.

Fast food chains are a perfect example of distributing highly processed food. Many of their products have exactly the same size, shape, and color. In certain restaurants, there are so many preservatives in the food that they can be left for *over a year* without growing mold or even deteriorating. Think again next time you eat at any fast food restaurant. **If at all possible, don't buy highly packaged or similar shaped foods, and get rid of the ones that pack your kitchen shelves.**

Toss the Temptations

Many times when we are stressed or just don't know what to do, we turn to old habits of comfort—like that ex you swore you'd never talk to again. How much good did that ever do? None. So stay away from them. Food is no different. Just because you think it might "solve" a temporary problem doesn't mean it will.

Whenever you are hungry, stressed, or whatever, you will probably eat what is accessible. Sweets destroy diets and increase the risk of diabetes, heart disease, and other long-term health issues. Perhaps you don't crave sweet foods or eat sweets when stressed. You may prefer breads or salty foods, but both salty and carb-loaded foods are also easy to binge eat. High sugar, high salt, and high carb foods quickly degrade your valiant effort to eat healthy.

"Kill the craving with healthier alternatives."

Don't let these unhealthy foods develop into addictions. Eliminate them before they do any more damage.

While completely removing them is the best method for controlling your unhealthy eating habits, keeping healthier alternatives that still crunch that craving is essential.

I call this craving the "forbidden fruit syndrome." When someone tells you that you can't eat something, what do you want to eat? That exact thing. Therefore, we must be prudent when it comes to our trigger foods. Don't let the mentality of "not having" certain foods dominate you. Kill the craving by enjoying a healthier alternative.

Food Dating Questions

The primary reason for introducing these five methods is to help you get a basic understanding of which foods to be wary. The better idea you have of the hazards, the more likely you are to stay away from them. These methods will change how you look at food and reduce the chances of eating junk that you shouldn't touch in the first place.

Reduce or eliminate the opportunity and temptation of unhealthy foods by following these five methods. They are some of the most important aspects of a healthy long-term food relationship.

Now, it's time for action. Clean out that kitchen. Let's see how well you score with our five steps for improving your food choices. Did you really break up with the bad and take the necessary steps for finding food relationship success?

Which foods on your typical grocery list now endanger your food relationship?

Are you surprised by how many unhealthy/processed foods you own?

List the foods that you removed from your cabinets, pantry, etc.

Briefly write down your emotions during this process.

Did you have the willpower to remove your vice foods? Why or why not?

Are you able to come up with healthy alternatives for every food that you removed?

Are these methods easy to follow? Why or why not?

If you have cleaned out the bad, you have taken one of the largest and most difficult steps towards a simple and healthy food relationship.

The breakup is the hardest step to starting a new future. Removing unhealthy foods from your cabinets and getting them out of your life is difficult. However, instead of mourning a relationship that was no good for you in the first place, start to focus your energy on the relationships that really matter.

You've figured out which foods you need to stay away from, so now let's talk about healthy options, navigating the grocery aisles, and which foods help you develop long-term relationships that are worth keeping.

8 Simple Steps to Long-Term Relationship Success

Buying the right food and making sure you eat a well-balanced diet are the most important parts of a long-term relationship. However, the temptations of vending machines, fast food, sweets, and events can quickly shove many of those well-planned eating habits to the back of our minds. How do we address these everyday struggles? By understanding what we actually need so that we have the freedom and insight to make the best choices.

Maybe it's been awhile since you were on the food dating scene, and you've grown accustomed to your old grocery list. Don't be nervous about trying new, healthier options. Even if you've had a bad track record with falling for lousy food or not realizing a poor choice until it's too late, this section will help you understand what to look for in a new relationship and how to be victorious day-in and day-out.

What Should My Calorie Intake Be?

One of the most important aspects of any food relationship is how much you eat every day. Knowing this is best accomplished by keeping track of what you eat, commonly known as counting calories. Because honest relationships are best, think of tracking your calories as an accountability partner.

There are many different factors that go into the calorie equation, but it is primarily centered on your current weight, age, activity level, and goals for gaining or losing weight. For most individuals, the median calorie intake per day is around 2,000 calories. This keeps things simple when nutrition labels are concerned because it allows every food to be measured by the same scale. However, just because that is the median intake for most does not mean it is your ideal number.

Instead of worrying about complicated equations to figure out your daily calorie intake, we are going to keep it simple. There are three easy ways to cut the fluff and still find your calorie intake.

First Method of Calorie Counting: Using a Food-Tracking App

Go to your app store on your cell phone and simply type in "food tracker app." Follow the prompts and you are ready to go. Many of the apps only require that you type in your weight, activity level, and other basic information. As soon as you enter the information, it will give you a calorie number. This is the easiest and most effective method. Some of the most popular food tracking apps are Myfitnesspal, Myplate, and Lose It.

If you want to lose weight, reduce your calories
by 300-500 a day.
If you want to gain weight, increase your calories
by 300-500 a day.

Second Method of Calorie Counting: The Multiplier Method

If you need a good approximation (within 100 calories or so), the multiplier method works well. Take your current weight and just multiply. If you know how many calories you burn during exercise, then it will help account for your calories during the day. "Active" is considered working a manual labor job or burning roughly 300+ calories per day during exercise. "Not Active" is for jobs that require little or no exertion (desk jobs).

Active / Non-Active & Goals	Formula Weight (lbs) x Value Weight (kg) x Value	Recommended Daily Calorie Intake
Not Active & Weight Loss	Weight (lb.) x10.15 Or Weight (kg) x 22.3	
Not Active & Weight Maintenance	Weight (lbs.) x12 Or Weight (kg) x 26.4	
Active & Weight Loss ½ lb. / ¼ kg per Week	Weight (lbs) x14 Or Weight (kg) x 30.8	
Active & Weight Maintenance	Weight (lbs) x16 Or Weight (kg) x 35.2	
Active & Weight Gain of ½ lb. / ¼ kg per Week	Weight (lbs) x18 Or Weight (kg) x 39.6	

Third Method of Calorie Counting: The Golden Calorie Method

There are 3,500 kcal in a pound of body fat, so if you want to lose weight at a safe rate, simply knowing how many calories you take in a day is important. One week of cutting out 500 extra calories a day equals 1 pound of fat. By the way, one extra "snack" a day can easily equal 500 calories or more.

Based on the previous formulas, you should now have an idea of how many calories you should personally be taking in every day. **If you are burning more than you are taking in, you will lose weight and vice versa.** It is really that easy. The hard part is being patient enough to eat the right foods at the right time.

Safe weight loss is about 1 pound (0.45 kg) per week. When changing your diet, you will most likely experience drastic weight loss for the first couple months, followed by a plateau period. This is where exercise and continual healthy eating habits are most important. Stick with it, and you will get the results you want.

What is a Well-Rounded Diet?

Dynamic and fun relationships always keep things fresh and new. Your food relationship should be the same. After you determine what should be your calorie intake, make it a goal to meet that number with a variety of quality proteins, fruits, vegetables, and fiber **every day**. Constant variations of healthy food equates to a "well-rounded diet."

The variety in your diet is best reflected by your "end of the day summary" in a food tracking app. Many of these apps automatically set up specific percentage ranges for you and are customizable depending on your goals. If you can stick to similar values every day, your chances of success will greatly increase.

BREAKDOWNS	PROTEIN %	CARBOHYDRATE %	FAT %
THE "TYPICAL"	15-35	55-65	10-15
THE "BALANCE"	33	33	33
THE "LEAN GAINER"	40	30	30

The recommended breakdown is the "Typical," as it is more flexible and allows for the easiest transition from a "non-diet" centered lifestyle. You will gradually find what percentages work best for you after about 2-3 weeks of tracking. The "Balance" and "Lean Gainer" are for those who already know how many calories they intake and can manage them effectively. Diets with higher protein percentages are typically combined with resistance training programs and should be recommended by your doctor, dietician, or nutritionist first.

Calorie counting is not necessary; however, calorie counting does give you a better idea of what foods you are eating, of what they

Recalibrate your calorie intake every 5 (2.5 kg) pounds you lose or gain to stay on track and not overeat.

consist, and whether you should eat more or less throughout the day. Basic calorie tracking also helps keep you accountable, whether you are trying to lose, gain, or maintain weight. Once you have tracked your food for a period of 5-6 months, you will most likely be able to determine if you have eaten too much or too little, and you will know what foods sabotage those numbers.

How Much Should I Be Eating?

Successful relationships rely on constant affirmation. If you hear from your loved one only once a day, problems will probably arise; the better the communication, the better the understanding, and fewer the problems. Similarly, the more in-tune you are with your body, the more your food relationship will improve. This is especially true if you find yourself constantly hungry, tired, or moody. It's time to prioritize meals and change how much and when you eat.

You should try to eat three full meals a day, with two or three healthy snacks a day. It may sound like too much, but starting to get hungry is your body signaling that it needs fuel. Eating healthy food more often helps boost your metabolism and provide your body with plenty of essential vitamins and nutrients. Eating quality foods, such as lean proteins (meats with less fat)

The term "full meal," doesn't mean binging or eating more than you should. Stick to your numbers. It's easy to overeat at every meal, so slow down and enjoy your food.

and complex carbohydrates (whole wheat/grain products), throughout the day is key to satiation.

Basic Breakdown of a 2,000 kcal daily diet

Here are just a few different calorie breakdowns of the thousands that are possible. Different intakes will vary on work schedule, life events, and habits.

Breakdown One

Breakfast	400 calories
Snack	300 calories
Lunch	500 calories
Snack	200 calories
Dinner	600 calories

Breakdown Two

Breakfast	300 calories
Snack	200 calories
Lunch	700 calories
Snack	100 calories
Dinner	700 calories

Breakdown Three

Breakfast	350 calories
Snack	150 calories
Lunch	850 calories
Snack	150 calories
Dinner	500 calories

Stages of Love (aka Breakfast, Lunch, and Dinner)

Our moods change throughout the day based on a variety of circumstances. One of the best ways to boost our energy, improve our mood, and increase productivity is by eating the right foods at the right times. These simple tips can help make or break your food relationship. Although it may sound simple, we often forget how important a single meal is.

Breakfast

Waking up next to your significant other and screaming insults is an absolutely terrible way to start the day—not to mention, treat someone. The same goes for your body. Don't insult your body by feeding it unhealthy foods first thing in the morning.

Breakfast should be the most important meal of the day. It gets your body ready for the upcoming hours and determines what nutritional course you are going to travel. Society's choices for breakfast are typically higher carbohydrate meals like cereal, oatmeal, breads, or whichever biscuit sounds tasty in the fast food line. There is little thought about what is consumed, as long as it alleviates the after-sleep hunger, is quick, and convenient. All this convenience and on-the-go eating can be disastrous for your food relationship. Starting off the day with high-sugar/high carbohydrate foods won't keep you full for very long, which will lead to overeating, fat storage, and hunger later in the day. **Incorporating lean proteins into our diets (especially at**

breakfast) will help balance daily intakes, increase meal satiety, and decrease hunger throughout the day.

In addition to unhealthy breakfast foods, we typically over-caffeinate with coffee or energy drinks in the morning. Coffee and other caffeinated drinks act as diuretics, which increase the risk of dehydration through excess urination of water and other nutrients. Ironically, instead of preparing our bodies for the upcoming day, we often do the complete opposite and sabotage it. Think twice next time before you choose your breakfast.

What are some easy ways to eat a healthier breakfast?

> Think about what you will cook/prepare the night before.
> Incorporate a lean protein into your breakfast (eggs, Greek yogurt, turkey sausage/bacon, etc.).
> Drink a large glass of water when you wake up. Water helps rehydrate you and will most likely ease any stomach discomfort for those who are not used to eating food in the mornings. It also aids in digestion and weight loss, so why not start off early?
> Think about foods that are easy and quick to make (natural peanut butter toast with a banana, fresh fruit in Greek Yogurt or Low Fat Cottage Cheese, eggs, egg tortilla, quiche—prepared the night before).
> Try new things. With the lists in this book, you should have plenty of options for the foods that are healthy and tasty!

Lunch

Lunch should be a continuation of breakfast, with some added calories and variety. Unfortunately, lunch is the most common meal eaten at work or on-the-go. This makes lunch the meal that is most susceptible to fast food chains and restaurants. Poor planning the night before or impulse decisions when deciding on a restaurant will quickly ruin your daily caloric intake.

Be cognizant while ordering meals, and stick to the guidelines for restaurants (as explained in the upcoming pages). If you didn't bring your lunch, go online and review the menu for your restaurant pick of the day. This will help you choose a healthier option before stepping through the doors.

If you typically struggle with energy before or after lunch, eat clean carbohydrates, such as vegetables, non-processed breads, and fruits—and don't forget about water! Remember that lunch is typically your half-way point in the day, so don't go hungry and make sure to provide yourself with plenty of fuel to finish strong.

What should I think about when eating lunch?

- Try to make your own food and bring it to work.
- Consider meal prepping. It saves money and time when compared to eating out—and is healthier as well.
- Try to incorporate more greens into your meal.
- If a restaurant is severely limited on the amount of greens they offer on the menu, eat somewhere else.
- Salads with chicken or whole-wheat subs/sandwiches are great healthy lunches. Tuna and chicken salad are also easily portable and tasty.
- Prepare or buy a meal centered on your activities later in the day (manual labor occupations or post-work exercise needs higher carbohydrate and water consumption).

Dinner

When we think of romance, candlelit dinners with tables full of scrumptious food come to mind. While this may be the most picturesque meal of the entire day, it is the most detrimental to our dietary goals.

Dinner is often the largest meal of the day, typically eaten in the evening. This gives our bodies only a small window of time to break down large food portions before we go to sleep. When we go to bed, our bodies still burn calories but at a slower rate. Therefore, if we binge eat at night (excess eating, desserts, and/or alcoholic beverages), then we not only lose a day's worth of healthy eating but also the excess calories that are not burned are turned into fat. Don't make this mistake. Enjoy your food in moderation, and plan on an earlier dinner time. Try to stick to a similar calorie intake as your lunch, if not slightly less.

Fortunately, many restaurant dinner menus are diverse, giving you more options and opportunities to make better choices. **Consistently choose healthy options, and your weight goals will be achieved before you know it.**

One of the greatest influences on your eating habits at any restaurant is how hungry you are before getting there. If you go to a restaurant excessively hungry, you will most likely overeat. Skipping the appetizers and reducing your bread intake prior to the main course are key considerations for keeping your food commitment in check. You can also split a meal with a friend, which cuts the large portion of food—and the bill—in half. With a little bit of patience and planning, your food relationship will strengthen when it is being tested in environments such as these.

Snacks

We've covered all of the meals throughout the day, but what about snacks? If you are going to stay on track with a healthy diet, you need quality snacks. As we expend energy throughout the day, we are tempted to grab whatever is close and convenient to "hold us over." However, these impulse snacks can lead to diet disaster. One small dessert or bag of chips can throw your entire regime off track and negate all of your exercising for that day. For instance, a single scoop of ice cream contains about 150 calories, and a snack-sized bag of Lay's potato chips contains 160 calories. How often do we eat only one scoop of ice cream or just one small bag of chips? Rarely. Find what foods you love the most, and figure out which ones would be great additions throughout the day.

A healthy snack contains anywhere from 100-300 calories, consisting of a lean protein, complex carbohydrate, and/or healthy fat.

Nuts are especially a great snack throughout the day. Just be cautious of their high calorie count. Portion out the amount you will eat before digging in the bag.

Top Recommended Nuts

TYPE OF NUT	CALORIES	PROTEIN (G)	FAT (G)
ALMOND	163	6	14
PISTACHIO	59	5.8	12.9
CASHEW	157	5.2	12.4
WALNUT	178	4.2	17.5
BRAZIL	186	4.1	18.8

20 Recommended Snacks
Almonds / Pistachios
Apple / Banana with Peanut Butter
Baked Sweet Potato
Can of Tuna / Tuna and Crackers
Carrots and Hummus
Citrus Fruit
Cottage Cheese
Edamame
Hard/Soft-boiled Eggs
Kale Chips
Mozzarella Cheese Stick
PB&J on 100% Whole Wheat Bread
Peanut Butter with whole wheat crackers
Plain Greek Yogurt (add peanut butter for flavor)
Protein Bar (lower sugar and higher protein)
Protein Shake
Protein Trail Mix
Sliced Avocado
Soy Nuts
Sunflower Seeds

Portion Sizes & Basic Eating Habits

Oftentimes we associate binge eating with unhealthy foods. However, it is still possible to binge on healthy foods. When it all comes down to it, too many calories is just unhealthy. With an excess of calories, no matter how good or how bad the food is, you will gain weight.

Unfortunately, what is now perceived as a "normal" portion is much more than you need. Portion sizes have grown over the years and gotten out of hand. From 20 years ago, similar servings, calories, and food portions have doubled and even tripled, and it is wreaking havoc on our waistlines and health. These "regular" portions have distorted our thinking of what meal size we need.

If you are over 40 years old, the meals you used to eat when you were 20 years old have probably drastically changed along with your body. Your metabolism has slowed down, and the portions have gotten bigger—two things that work against you. You must be even more cognizant when it comes to eating.

Fortunately, no matter your age, these guidelines will help you avoid nutritional pitfalls next time you eat:

1. Center your meal on a lean protein: This should be about the *size of your palm* (fish, turkey, beef, fish, wild game, etc).
2. Vegetables: This should be about the size of *your closed fist*.
3. Carbohydrates: This should be about the size of *1-cupped hand or less* (breads, potatoes, rice).
4. Fats: These should be able the size *of your thumb* (butters, oils, nuts).
5. Don't overeat: It is better to start with less food on your plate to avoid the likelihood of overeating or binge eating.
6. The better food you eat during your meal, the more satisfied you will be once it is over.
7. Don't feel as though you have to clean your plate.
8. Stick to your daily dietary goals and caloric intake.
9. Eat slowly. Give your body time to tell you it is full.
10. Eat small dessert portions slowly. After 10-15 minutes, you will be less likely to eat more dessert.

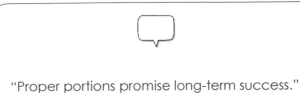

"Proper portions promise long-term success."

Still Hungry?

What should you do if you are still hungry after eating a meal or even a snack? This can get complicated very quickly (based on foods eaten, timing, liquid intake, energy used, etc.), so we should stick to this simplified strategy to attack hunger:

> **Step 1:** Wait 10 Minutes
> **Step 2:** Ask yourself, "am I really hungry, just craving, bored, or overeating?"
> **Step 3:** If you feel hungry but not enough to eat an entire meal, it is probably best to wait a little longer until your next full meal.

Don't give into the nagging impulses, especially if you have just eaten plenty of food—maybe even plus some—in the past hour or two. Drink water instead to crunch that craving. If you begin grazing non-stop throughout

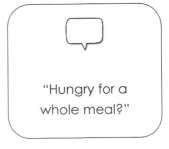

"Hungry for a whole meal?"

the day, it doesn't matter if it's the healthiest thing is the world, you will more than likely overeat and begin stacking on unnecessary pounds.

Long-Term Commitment Questions.

Based on your calorie counting phone app, what is the recommended daily intake? Compare this to your number for the Multiplier Method.

Are you active or inactive? What are some ways you can become more active?

How many calories do you typically eat during breakfast, lunch and dinner? Snacks?

What are the typical percentages that you typically eat? (Protein, Carbohydrates, and Fats)

What foods do you typically overeat or binge on?

What is a good snack that you can start eating at least once a day?

Meal Prepping and Why You Should Consider It

Our lives are often chaotic, making it hard to eat healthy. This is where meal prepping saves us. Typically we stereotype bodybuilders and the hardcore workout fanatics as those carrying around Tupperware containers of food—and eating what seems like ten times a day—but in reality, meal prepping is for everyone. Whether you want to gain weight, lose weight, or maintain weight, you should strongly consider meal prepping if you want to strengthen your commitment to eating healthy.

The Love-Hate Relationship with Meal Prepping

People primarily prep meals to adhere to their daily recommended calorie intake. Another major benefit of prepping is if it is time to eat or you are hungry, just throw the meal in the microwave, and BAM—you're done! There's no time to be tempted by vending machines or fast food fries. To get started, you only need some food containers and a couple sets of utensils. And, there's no worry about overeating or undereating because you've already precisely portioned meals at the beginning of the week.

At first, meal prepping may seem constraining or a hassle, but in reality meal prepping gives you freedom. Preparing the meals typically only takes one or two days a week, and because you are preparing the food, you can pick the kinds of protein, vegetables, and carbs that you want and need. If you have a specific taste, you can add spices or sauces unique to your liking. If you know what you will be doing for the week ahead, you can prepare your meals accordingly. If you need more carbs or protein than usual, you don't have to rely on hoping to find a healthy restaurant or finding the time to fight traffic. All the work has already been done.

Meal prepping also makes logging your food easier, as you can replicate your meals every day. Anytime there is a deviation from your plan, it's easy to tell where you went astray.

While the positives outweigh the negatives of meal prepping, there are a few important things to consider before you go buy all the food. With only one or two preparation days, plan on spending two or three hours each of those days cooking, cutting, and packing. If you were to map out the amount of time spent cooking every afternoon or waiting in the fast food line, meal prepping would still save you time. Just consider that now you need a concentrated block of time to prepare everything.

The cost of buying a supply of healthy food all at one time may seem expensive at checkout. With this in mind, think about all the money you spend every week at restaurants. It is easy to spend 10-15 dollars on just one meal. Add up all of those meals throughout the week, and the money you spend on quality food at the store pales in comparison to what you will get at a restaurant. With meal prepping, you also know how everything is prepared, what ingredients are in it, and how many calories it contains.

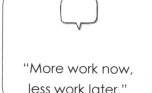

"More work now, less work later."

Social settings and peer pressure can be another struggle of meal-prepping. If you are not willing to stick to a specific meal plan and would rather eat out, meal prepping may not be for you. Your peers are probably not as driven as you are when it comes to reforming their food relationships. **Remember it's *your***

relationship, not theirs. Peer pressure and the avoidance of certain foods or restaurants may be difficult to address depending on your occupation or trade; however, if you are able to eat your meal before going out to eat, you will consume fewer calories at the restaurant and be more likely to stick to your daily calorie goals.

Perhaps the greatest complaint about meal prepping is the tendency to become boring and mundane very quickly, especially since you eat many of the same meals day-after-day. This is why it is important to mix up your spices, seasonings, and marinades often.

If you feel as though packing meal-after-meal in containers is silly or impractical, then make a larger quantity of food than normal when cooking at home. The excess can be left-overs for the next few days. While eating leftovers is anything but new, it can help break up the monotony of eating the same meal two or three times a day.

There are many different ways you can prep meals. The possibilities are endless when it comes to food combinations, so pick the ones you like and that match your dietary goals.

For instance: "Mason Jar Meals" are another great idea for meal prepping that typically caters better towards fresh fruits and vegetables.

Meal Prep Construction

This is the basic construction for your meals. I highly recommend adding a variety of meats, vegetables, and carbs to keep things interesting throughout the week. To start, divide up the food according to your daily percentages and your daily calorie intake. This will help you to determine what ratios are most appropriate for your containers.

1. Pick one lean protein.
2. Pick one fresh/frozen vegetable.
3. Pick a complex carbohydrate.
4. Determine your favorite sauces and spices.
5. Prepare foods and cook according to your tastes.
6. Divide up meats and vegetables. Do this for each specific meal.
7. Divide the protein, vegetable, and carbohydrate evenly amongst the containers.
8. Enjoy.

Foods for Meal Prepping
Lean Meats – Turkey, Fish, Chicken, Beef, Venison, Tofu
Broccoli / Cauliflower
Rice – Brown, White and Yellow
Green Beans
Quinoa
Potatoes – Sweet, White, Red
Hard Boiled Eggs
Peppers

Meal Prepping Challenge

What are your nutritional goals?

Do you need more structure in your eating habits? If so, where can you adjust your daily routine to accommodate?

How much time do you have for lunch? Do you feel rushed?

List five options for each of the following: meats, vegetables, fruits, and carbohydrates. These are good options to consider while making your meals for the week.

How much time are you willing to spend preparing food this week?

Fast Food, Restaurants, and Eating Out

Often the most difficult aspect of any food relationship takes place outside of the kitchen and grocery store. These temptations present themselves in an abundance of sit-down restaurants, fast-food restaurants, street vendors, and social events.

We are lured in by fancy signs, marketing campaigns, online reviews, and well, just being really hungry. Even when restaurants aren't marketing themselves visually, they often lure you through various aromas, despite your will to resist. Walk through the mall and be bombarded with fantastic fragrances coming from the cookie, donut, and pretzel stands. We are constantly surrounded by temptations.

Why do we crave fast food? Why do certain smells trigger our hunger? The answer is quite simple. Our brains push the reward button every time we see, hear, or smell something that we have enjoyed in the past. The carbs, sugars, fats, and salts associated with fast food, dessert, and other nutritionally empty foods activate the reward center in our brain. This causes a release of feel good chemicals (dopamine) in our body. Our brain's desire to eat these reward foods can quickly cause an addiction if we are not careful. Fast food is higher in fats and salts, which not only add inches to our waistlines but also increase our chances of developing health risks, directly destroying a healthy food relationship.

Fast food and convenient food also appeals to our comfort levels. We are creatures of comfort and often find relief in not having to put forth any effort in preparing our food, let alone think about the ramifications that come with poor choices. What sounds easier: Having someone make your food or making it yourself? **Of course it always sounds better to be waited on**

and not put any effort into making a meal, but comfort food can quickly become disastrous to your relationship. Complacency with nutrition is like staying in bad relationship. It doesn't benefit either party and is merely prolonging the inevitable—a breakup.

When you order food, you don't know anything about the ingredients, the preparation methods, how long it has been stored in the back, and what the actual calories are. You can always estimate the calories based on your food tracking apps, but the absolute best option is to be selective in your decisions on where and what you eat.

Here are some simple and healthy tips to remember how to stay on track, even when you are out and about but have to eat something:

1. **Ask yourself**: Is the restaurant known for having any healthy foods? Sorry, but pizza, chips, beer, and fried foods don't count as "healthy."

2. **Go with the** "Healthy Option," "Fresh Menu," "Lower calorie," or something similar if available.

3. **Check the calories for what you are about to eat.** Look at the calories on the menu, and if not available, look them up in your food app. If the menu doesn't have the calorie breakdowns, ask if there is a menu that has them listed.

4. **Order the grilled and baked options.** Stay away from "covered," "smothered," "fried," "creamy," "crusted," "cheesy," "breaded," and "crispy," as they often will spike your calories and increase the amount of fat and salt.

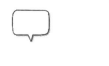

"If it covers food, watch out."

5. **Salads are a great meal.** Just stick with a lite dressing or vinaigrette, skip the croutons, and add a lean protein like chicken or strip steak.

6. **Drinks:** Go for a water, water with lemon or lime, tea (unsweetened), sports drink (PowerAde or Gatorade), or house coffee (drip or French press).

7. **Stick with whole wheat, wheat, or flat breads when ordering.** Limit appetizer breads, as they can ruin your entire meal and caloric intake for the day.

8. **Limit condiments.** Condiments are high in calories, salt, fat, and preservatives. Just 1 container of Zax Sauce from Zaxby's restaurant is 240 calories!

9. **Consider portion sizes.** Most serving sizes are way too big. Order from the kids menu or split a dish with someone else at the table.

10. Higher quality food and better cooking techniques require fewer sauces. You get what you pay for.

11. **Don't be lazy**. There are *some* healthy options at almost every restaurant, but it may take some digging to find them. It is worth it.

12. **If you must indulge in dessert, choose low calorie options.** If those aren't available, choose frozen yogurt or split the dessert with everyone. Limit yourself when eating desserts, as they are major "calorie bombs."

As a side note, try to avoid any trip inside a gas station. They are filled with nothing but unhealthy foods and beverages. When it comes to food, there should only be three things that are bought in a gas station: water, coffee, and fruit.

**Recommended
Healthy Fast Food
Chains**
Chipotle
Panera Bread
Chick-Fil-A
Subway
Jason's Deli

Surviving Holidays and Big Life Events without De-Railing Your Relationship

Each relationship has unique challenges. The holidays and special events are one of the greatest nutritional challenges you can face, so be aware during these momentous occasions.

Almost every holiday throughout the year calls for tons of food. Your mouth may water when even think about your favorite holiday dishes. While your palate may get to enjoy a variety of foods and drinks, these should be approached with caution and patience.

The holidays are known to add inches to your waistline because we have a tendency to binge eat and graze on snacks all day long, day after day. This is especially true during Thanksgiving and Christmas, where desserts and other treats are plentiful. So how do you keep your food relationship simple and healthy when being confronted with such a smorgasbord of food?

Before

If you know you are going to a family gathering or event where you anticipate eating calorie-dense foods (pastas, breads, desserts, etc.) you should:

1. Not starve yourself before arriving, as this will likely lead to binge eating.
2. Drink plenty of water before arriving. Water helps keep you hydrated, curb your hunger, and prevent overeating before the main meal arrives. It can also help prevent a hangover the next day if you're drinking alcohol.
3. Eat a lean protein snack before arriving.
4. Exercise first thing in the morning to get a start on countering the excess calories likely to follow. Cardio exercises like running, biking, and swimming are great options for burning calories.
5. If you will be joining a potluck dinner or something similar, bring a healthier dish that can be a fall back.
6. Keep in mind how many calories you plan on contributing to liquid calories (juice, wine, beer, liquor, soda/pop, lattes, etc.), and stick to that number.

During

Events and holidays only come once a year, so enjoy them and the food that comes with them. To avoid going overboard though, here are a few pointers to keep in mind:

1. Enjoy a variety of food but put smaller portions of each kind on your plate.
2. Large servings of calorie dense foods, like potatoes and pastas, swamp your calories for the day and will give you that overly full feeling in no time.
3. Eat slowly. It takes about 20 minutes for your stomach to relay to your brain that it is full. Give your body time to adjust to all the food you are eating.
4. Look up the various foods that you will be eating in your food tracking apps. That will help direct your selections.
5. If you plan on eating dessert, save some room for it.

After

We all know that dessert is an integral part of celebrations, so if we are going to take part in the dessert, let's be smart about it:

1. If there are multiple desserts, pick one or several small pieces (or slivers) of each that equate to one piece.
2. Go for desserts with fruit, real fruit.
3. Eat slowly—again. If anything you eat throughout an entire day can wreck your diet, dessert are it.
4. Instead of having a second piece of dessert, accompany the single piece with a glass of milk or a cup of coffee.
5. Try not eating dessert too close to bedtime. Allot for about 3+ hours if at all possible before you doze off for the night.

Cheat Meals

Okay, so what exactly are "cheat meals," and are they good? A cheat meal is a meal when you basically say, "I'm eating whatever I want." This can be seen as a selfish treat in the form of food while on a diet or eating clean. Cheat meals can be an acceptable release, but they can become bad very quickly. They can quickly lead to overeating and should be considered dangerous when trying to mend a broken food relationship.

If you have a tendency to binge eat, cheat meals are risky. Your risk is low if you can control your eating to one cheat meal every 5-8 days. Now, keep in mind that **I did not say a *cheat day*.** A cheat day is a definite way to sabotage your entire diet and throw off weeks of effort. Overeating unhealthy foods for three meals can easily add 3-5 lbs. to the scale.

If you are going to have a cheat meal, make it something that you really love; however, try sticking to your calorie intake for the day and getting a workout in beforehand. It may sound like a pain, but **once you change your perspective and realize that you can literally have your cake and eat it too, it is actually freeing.**

Keep in mind that you started this journey for a reason. Don't throw away your progress over one meal or one day. When you eat poorly, the person you cheat on is yourself. Thinking long-term will help alleviate the urge to overeat.

Diets and Detoxes

Fad diets are everywhere. You see and hear all about the latest diets on social media, infomercials, and television. Each of them claim to change your life by melting away the pounds and ridding your body of all the unhealthy toxins. You would think they are the ultimate "simple and healthy food relationship," but in reality they often steer you down paths of fluctuating weight, spending too much money, and still not getting results you really need. The likelihood of long-term adherence to any of the diets out there is also rare. This should be a signal of caution.

Anytime a diet is difficult to implement on a long-term basis, it typically has a weak foundation. Weak foundations may include things like eliminating entire food groups (such as carbs or fat), buying powders, buying pre-prepped meals, buying food that comes in containers, or mandating abstinence from certain foods containing "x" or "y" ingredients. Believe it or not, our bodies need a variety of foods from every food group. The secret is in portion control and food quality.

If you want to get on the right path, the only "diet" you should think about is one that consists of *all* food groups: quality vegetables, lean proteins, and whole grains.

Out of the hundreds of diets, there are only a couple good "diets": DASH Diet and Mediterranean Diet. Although I don't recommend any specific diet other than healthy eating, the DASH Diet and the Mediterranean Diet are both scientifically based and have proven to be sustainable over several years. Each diet has its own attributes that should give you good meal ideas for a variety of occasions.

The DASH Diet

The DASH Diet is one of the top-recommended diets on the market. It is recommended by The National Heart, Lung and Blood Institute, The American Heart Association, and The Dietary Guidelines for Americans. It is founded on the science of being healthier from the inside out—not just focusing on outward appearance.

The DASH Diet prioritizes proper amounts of sodium, nutrients, and vitamins. Keeping these things in specific ranges helps to reduce the likelihood of long-term health issues, such as hypertension (high blood pressure), cholesterol, diabetes, and heart disease. After all, DASH stands for "Dietary Approaches to Stop Hypertension."

Expect to eat lean meats like fish and poultry, plenty of vegetables, fruits, whole grains, nuts, and beans. The emphasis for this diet is an overall healthy body, not massive amounts of weight loss. This diet is not an overnight change but worth considering for long-term adherence and heart health.

The Mediterranean Diet

The Mediterranean Diet is one that has gained popularity over the years, as it contains many dietary similarities to those recommended by the American Heart Association. The diet has been around for over 20 years and has been shown to reduce the risk of mortality in those associated with it long-term. It not only incorporates lean meats, vegetables, fruits, and whole grains but also encourages the use of olive oil and some occasional wine.

The amount of dietary fat is slightly higher from nuts and olive oil than in the DASH Diet, but they are still within healthy levels. The Mediterranean Diet is known for recommending regular exercise and reducing the consumption of red meats to only a couple times a month, while fish and poultry are key staples. Butter is also eliminated and substituted with olive oil, adding a flare of spontaneity with the addition of extra oils and wine.

The Alkaline and Ketogenic Diets

The Alkaline Diet and Ketogenic Diets are currently booming with social media coverage. These diets primarily focus on limiting carbohydrate consumption, while increasing protein and fat intake to help drop tons of weight.

The Alkaline and Ketogenic Diets claim to burn fat once the body reaches a state of alkalosis. This state of alkalosis occurs from constantly eating foods that contain no carbohydrates, causing your body to tap into fat stores. This is most commonly seen from test strips monitoring your pH levels. If you turn the test strip a certain color, you are "in the fat burning zone."

Ironically, our body's pH levels are constantly alkalotic. Our blood levels are slightly above the neutral level around 7.35-7.45. While some foods do raise our pH levels, we should avoid a diet that is completely based on that. After all, our urine pH and blood pH levels are significantly different. Our bodies are intricate and extremely proficient in maintaining a healthy environment for daily functions. Trying to chemically offset the body's system is not a good foundation for a diet.

Long-term adherence is also extremely difficult for these diets. They are hard to adapt for most occasions, and they can become expensive. Remember, any program that completely restricts any aspect of your diet through the elimination of food categories makes long-term application challenging and may not give your body all the necessary nutrients that it needs.

Although these diets are difficult to maintain, they do encourage the regular consumption of better foods such as lean meats and vegetables. If you are looking for a quick-weight loss solution, make sure to consult your doctor or physician prior to initiating these programs. As enticing as trending diets may seem, a well-rounded diet with regular exercise will be your safest bet for healthy and sustainable weight loss.

Detoxes

We are continually assaulted with messages about how we need to cleanse our bodies, get more energy, and essentially "reset" our systems through detox programs. Detox stands for detoxification, implying that we have this huge deposit of contaminants in our bodies from the environment and foods we eat, which will harm our bodies and increase our chances of both short and long-term health issues. This is typically "remedied" through various supplements or fasts that thousands of companies offer for a "small" fee. Let me save you time and money, as well as from headaches, nausea, dehydration, electrolyte imbalances, and several other issues these programs may give you.

If we want to streamline our food relationship and continue to think long-term, then we must keep it simple and healthy. **Our bodies are amazing machines that are extremely efficient at detoxifying our systems**. Our kidneys, liver, skin, respiratory system, immune system, and gastrointestinal system all play crucial roles in preventing infections and removing them if they enter our bodies. Taking many of the supplements and products these various "health" companies offer can actually damage our systems.

Oftentimes, detox products sold are not regulated by the FDA and come with side-effects like dehydration, diarrhea, malnourishment, and nausea—often followed by rapid weight gain after cessation of the cleanse period. Many detox programs are expensive, require periods of hunger, and cause diarrhea, which can damage your gastrointestinal tract. A true detox is performed in a hospital setting when a patient has been exposed to unhealthy doses of drugs and/or other chemicals. A true detox is not drinking a powder or certain drink several times a day.

Here's the skinny on detox programs: **Stay away from them**. If you feel as though you need a boost in energy, want to lose weight fast, are dragging through the day, or can't concentrate, the problem is most likely associated with your daily habits—not extra contaminants that need to be flushed out of your system.

There are many things that "health" companies try to sell as products that we don't need. Some of these products create confusion about what we really need in our diets and how to live healthy. **Eat healthy, reduce stress and anxiety, and get more exercise.** These simple practices will help your body in the long run. Be patient. If you stick to healthy foods that are full of quality protein, fiber, and vitamins, then you won't need to worry about ingesting unregulated substances or participating in unhealthy habits to get you through the day.

"Detox detracts from how efficient our bodies are."

Long-Term Food Relationship Questions

How many calories should you be consuming a day?

Is your lifestyle considered "non-active?" What can you do to change this?

How are you going to order foods differently next time you visit a restaurant?

How many meals & snacks should you eat EVERY day?

Do you eat too quickly? Do you overeat? What are some ways you can easily remedy these food relationship blunders?

Which fad diets have you considered? Why?

> ➢ Stick to your Calorie goal for the day. If you know you are going to be eating higher Calorie foods, try to make room for them in your daily percentages.
> ➢ Watch your portion sizes. Less is better to start. Eat slowly.
> ➢ Try to eat 3 quality meals a day with 2-3 quality snacks between.
> ➢ Fast food and restaurant food is quick and convenient, but it can spell disaster for your diet and overall health.
> ➢ Be patient during the holidays. Pace yourself and don't overeat.
> ➢ Don't get sucked into fad diets or crazy detoxes. Stick with the only thing that works: a variety of healthy foods with healthy habits like adequate sleep, stress reduction, and exercise.

PART TWO:
Picking the Right Food

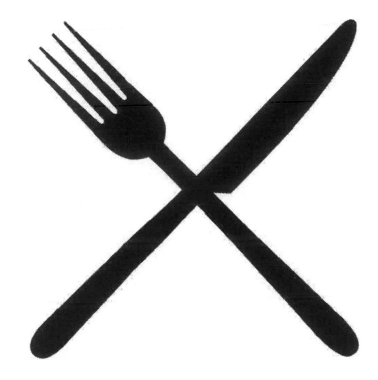

Getting Ready to Go Steady: Preparation for Shopping and Purchasing Your Food

Up to this point, we have gone over the steps for building and maintaining a healthy long-term food relationship. You can know your caloric intake and how many times you should eat a day, but if you don't actually buy or eat the foods that are beneficial, all your food knowledge is for nothing. This is where we talk food, real food—the stuff you will be buying year after year.

As we get closer to making our purchase decisions, keep in mind that going into any relationship blind and unprepared is unwise. If we want to go steady with the right food, then developing a needs and wants based shopping list *before* we go to the store is imperative. This list will help you streamline the shopping experience, avoid failure, and keep the momentum going.

Remember when we got rid of all those unnecessary items in your cabinets? Hopefully there is plenty of space now for healthy alternatives. If you completed this step, you are now ready to go shopping. If not, go back and get cleaning.

What Do You Want in Your Perfect Diet?

We can ask thousands of questions before heading to the store, but we must first consider the basics. Just like a date, we need to know where we are going, what time of year it is, and who or what is involved. The same goes for grocery shopping.

Questions to streamline creating a list may include: How many people am I shopping for? What are my nutritional goals? What are my family's (spouse's) nutritional goals?

Additional questions to develop a list that aids in accomplishing your nutritional goal should be: How many meals do I plan on cooking this week? Am I going to try and prepare any new dishes? What is my budget?

Once you answer these questions, cruising the aisles becomes much easier and faster.

For how many people are you shopping?

On what are your nutritional goals based (eating less, eating more)? Your spouse's? Family's?

How are you going to accommodate your goals AND the goals of your family members with the SAME foods?

How many home-cooked meals are you going to prepare? Do you have all of the necessary ingredients, spices, etc.?

What holidays, birthdays, or celebrations are in the next two weeks?

Where are you going to shop, and why?

What is the absolute maximum amount of money you are willing to spend on these groceries? Does this figure work with your monthly budget?

Now that you know what you are prepared for, it is time to start developing a grocery list. This is the biggest step in developing a healthy nutritional relationship.

Developing a Grocery List: What You Need for Your Perfect Diet

Your nutritional relationship is formed by the foods you put in your cart. You can make a great shopping list, but any deviation from the list can spell disaster. These deviations often stem from impulse decisions or uncertainty about healthy options. Various food commercials and food posts on social media tend to make things difficult as they tap into your cravings and can send you down a road of impulse eating. Removing these temptations will help you fight against poor decisions that you will regret later.

To develop a strong grocery list, we need to be informed and patient. Many of the items we think are healthy are actually the complete opposite. Marketing and packaging often obscures what is truly healthy. For instance, just because something mentions the words "diet," "fat-free," or "organic" does not necessarily indicate that it is better for you. Being informed about various foods empowers you to make better decisions.

Patience and long-term thinking is another key concept to developing a healthy grocery list. With this in mind, what you *need* to eat is not always what you *want* to eat. Although this may be an unfortunate fact, it branches into every other facets of life. If we only did what we want and never what we need, we would cease to exist. Eating healthy is a necessity.

Creating a strong and steady food relationship takes time and is not developed in a single day. However, because you have already established goals and answered the challenge questions, you are ready to start making the right purchases and become empowered through them. Your initial list may change because you are learning and changing it according to your needs.

Grocery List Necessity Questions

So far, we've discussed general guidelines and concepts for creating a flourishing food relationship, but before we go into the dirty details about specific foods, try your new skills by creating your own shopping list.

Make a shopping list *before* **you read the following section. Are any of the foods you wrote down ones to avoid based on the five rules discussed earlier (cleaning out your cabinets)? If so, what foods can you substitute for those?**

What foods are on your list that are not typically on your list?

Will you have the rights kinds of food for your family for the next week(s)?

If you feel a little uncertain about your shopping list and are wondering if the items actually measure up to what you deserve in a fulfilling nutritional life, don't worry. We'll revisit these questions at the end of the section. You will hopefully experience a change in thinking when you learn to avoid many of the supermarket deceptions. Think of this next section as a matchmaker, giving you only the best and most desirable foods to choose. By the time we reach the end, you'll be wondering why empty calories and fattening treats were ever appealing.

How to Make the First Move: Buying Your Groceries

There are many things to consider when buying groceries, especially when the aisles are stacked from top to bottom with countless options. So, let's narrow it down and make life a little easier.

Start by researching nearby stores that offer the best selection for your list. Search according to your current tastes, preferences, and needs. If you are looking for fresh vegetables then farmers' markets, stores known for organic produce, and even small stands on the side of the road may offer the best selection. If you are less picky or have no particular sense of direction, big box stores like Kroger, Wal-Mart, Safeway, Giant, and Publix may be good options.

Next, **remember the food you removed in the first place and why.** Use the 5 Rules for Cleaning out Your Cabinets to ask questions about items on your list:

1. Is it instant or microwaveable?
2. What's the expiration date?
3. Are there too many or unknown ingredients listed?
4. Is it highly packaged or perfectly shaped?
5. Have I eliminated sweets and craving foods?

Answering these five questions, you will more than likely be led to the perimeter of the store. **Sticking to the outside of the store is exactly what you want to create a solid foundation of foods.** The outskirts of the store consist primarily of vegetables, fruits, meat, and frozen foods. Many of the items on the rim of the store, typically, have shorter shelf lives. Based on what we covered earlier, this means they are healthier for you.

When you shop in the middle of the store (the top-to-bottom shelving aisles), it is best to be highly selective. Keep in mind that items in the inner aisles usually have longer shelf lives and typically contain more preservatives, artificial flavors, and artificial sweeteners.

A few items that are quality purchases in the middle of the store are canned goods (low/no sodium added), 100% whole-wheat pastas, breads, brown rice, dried beans, and some condiments.

Keep in mind that it is important to stick to your shopping list once you enter the grocery store. Also, avoid making a grocery list or going shopping while you are hungry or thirsty. Your purchases will be based more on your hunger and getting through the aisles quickly rather than on making smart decisions.

In order to make the best food decisions, it is important to individually address each of the primary food groups. While we cannot cover every food here, it is crucial to keep your goals and needs in mind while making your individual selections. "Quality over quantity" will be one of your best determining factors when trying to decide which option to pick.

Meat

Start with your meat selection, as it is a great way to condense time spent in the store and help you plan specific meals. Centering meals on protein is a great habit, as this helps make meal planning easier and increases satiety.

When you purchase meat, buy lean meats whenever possible. Lean meats contain less saturated fat and have higher protein content. Saturated fat is not good for your arteries, so it's best to introduce the least amount possible to your body.

Fish and venison are the absolute best picks for the highest amount of protein per serving, followed closely by chicken and turkey. Beef, pork, and lamb also have moderately high protein values but typically contain more fat per ounce. Unfortunately, only a few types of seafood and shellfish are recommended due to their high sodium and cholesterol levels. More processed meats like sausages, hot dogs, and bratwursts are not recommended at all due to their higher fat and sodium content.

The Debate: Grass Fed vs Grain-Fed cattle & Free-Range vs Cage-Free Chicken

There are many different ways to raise livestock, poultry, and fish, but which ways are the healthiest? Grass Fed vs Grain-Fed cattle, Free-Range vs Cage-Free chicken: Which one is healthier for your relationship? **When we think about eating healthy, we assume eating grass-fed beef or cage-free chicken are healthier choices, but this simply isn't true.**

These are hotly debated topics, as they are ethically controversial and involve multi-billion dollar corporations who are trying to compete with one another. When it comes down to what livestock or poultry you should eat, it should be founded on the *nutritional value, cost,* and *your own ethical stance.* These three things will help you determine what the best fit is for you and your budget.

When you are talking about the livestock industry in America, beef is the primary meat product. Most beef sold in the U.S. is either grain-fed or grass-fed. Grass-fed cattle tend to have a higher percentage of grass in their diets compared to that of strictly grain-fed cattle, whose diets incorporate a mixture of hay, grain, and corn. Grass-fed cattle are also associated with having more sanitary living conditions than that of grain-fed cattle. Many grain-fed cattle are contained in Concentrated Animal Feeding Operations (CAFO), which have been associated with unethical animal treatment and the use of unnecessary hormones and steroids.

Cattle's living conditions and dietary intake are the two primary factors that determine which type of beef is actually healthier. Grass-fed beef is said to have higher amounts of B vitamins, omega 3 fatty acids, and other minerals, but these claims cannot always be substantiated since the location of the cattle farms and their living conditions greatly vary from one region to the next.

In a multi-billion dollar industry, it is no surprise that many disagreements over which is healthier have arose, and there are multiple studies that produce conflicting data. In the end, ethics are the determining factor—even though grass-fed does appear to be slightly healthier.

Primary differences between grass-fed and grain-fed are also the price and the taste. Grass-fed is 2-3 times the price of grain-fed and is only found in select stores. Ironically, many people prefer the taste of grain-fed meats but choose grass-fed for ethical reasons or the minor difference in nutritional value.

Poultry is not very different than cattle when it comes to how they are raised. Even though poultry is marketed as free-range (having access to the outdoors) or cage-free (no cages), nearly every ounce of chicken and chicken egg sold comes from highly confined and overcrowded chicken houses. Large chicken companies have simply exploited the definitions of what free-range and cage-free should truly be. When you think of cage-free and free-range, you probably imagine chickens living freely in the fields, but this is simply not the case. Just like in the cattle industry, profit, not the treatment of animals, is the primary motivating factor.

Nutritionally speaking, if you buy "free-range" or "cage-free" eggs from any major company, they have virtually the same nutritional profile as that of regular caged chickens. Your absolute best bet is to buy from local farmers for eggs, chicken, and beef. **Buying locally is healthier for your body and your local community relationships**. If you cannot buy locally, simply stick with regular beef and chicken as there are virtually no differences except in price.

Chicken

Chicken is one of the leanest and most versatile meats you can buy. **Every ounce of chicken contains 8g of protein, no carbs, no sugar, and very little fat.** You can eat it during any meal and mix it in with almost anything. The meal options for chicken are endless.

Some of the most versatile and common cuts are chicken breasts and tenderloins. They are healthy in both the fresh and frozen options. If you buy fresh chicken but for some reason won't be able to finish it all in time, just throw it in the freezer and save it for later. If you are looking to skip out on cooking entirely or need a quick option, rotisserie chickens are the way to go. They are quick, easy, and often provide enough meat to feed a small family. Anytime you can feed the family a lean, healthy protein and make it thousands of different ways, you have found yourself a winner. These are just a couple of reasons why you should consider chicken several times a week.

Turkey

Another great meat selection is turkey. It's packed full of protein and contains virtually no fat. **An ounce of turkey (turkey breast) contains 40 calories, which packs 9.5g of protein, 1.2 carbs, and .5g of fat.** Whether it's your Thanksgiving turkey, ground turkey, or hand-sliced deli turkey, you can't go wrong.

Turkey is often so lean (ground turkey is typically 93% lean and 7% fat) that unless you add additional spices, sauces, or condiments, it can be dry and bland. This is typically why there is gravy on the Thanksgiving table or ketchup and mustard for turkey burgers. While the extra sauces and condiments can liven up turkey, they also increases the calories per serving. With the right spices and seasonings, you can keep the calorie count low and still enjoy a tasty meal—just go low on the sodium.

Top Recommended Turkey Picks
Hand sliced turkey breast
Ground turkey
Deli turkey

Another great thing about turkey is that it can help lower your cholesterol levels. Simply substitute it for any recipe that calls for ground beef. When walking the aisles, your eye might catch turkey bacon, but be cautious. This is not the same kind of substitute. Although it may appear a healthier option when compared to pork bacon, it is still high in sodium and saturated fat. It is not as high as pork bacon, but it is much more processed. Why do you think every slice of turkey bacon looks *exactly* the same?

Consider eating turkey two or three times a week. Once you get used to cooking with it, which isn't challenging because it's not that much different than ground beef, you will be reaping the benefits of a lean and tasty protein.

Deli meats

Deli meats can be a great go-to food when trying to eat healthy, save time, and mix things up. There are many cuts to choose from, so narrowing down which ones are the best is often difficult.

The first rule of deli meats is to stay away from the pre-packaged meats. Although the pre-packed meats allow for ease of purchase, they are often filled with more preservatives and sodium than the hand sliced deli counter options. Their lower prices and extended expiration dates are two good indicators of the additives they may contain. The best options are hand-sliced by the deli clerk. Both options though are still higher in sodium and preservatives than the true cuts of meat, so be cautious with your weekly consumption.

The lower sodium meats are the healthiest options; however, they do tend to lack some taste. Smoked or baked options typically contain more

Healthiest Deli Meats
Turkey
Roast Beef
Ham
Least Healthy Deli Meats
Bologna
Salami
Pastrami
Mortadella

flavor and only slightly bump up the calories. If you are looking for some interesting ways to mix up your deli meats, you can chop them up and put them on a salad, make a Panini, or add them to an egg omelet. There are countless ways to use deli meat, so enjoy the process of experimenting and having fun.

Beef and Steak

There are plenty of pros and cons to eating red meat, so let's keep it simple. **Red meat is a great source of protein, vitamin B, vitamin D, and minerals such as iron, zinc, and magnesium.** Beef is also unfortunately a source for saturated fat, which can lead to unhealthy cholesterol levels.

When trying to portion meat per person, an appropriate average of about ½ lb. (8 oz.) per grown male and 1/3 lb. (5 oz.) for a grown female. Whether you like steak rare or well-done, just be sure to cook it until the temperature is 160° F or 71° Celsius.

When you are buying ground beef, opt for the lean beef, which is typically sold with proportions of 93-94% lean and only 6-7% fat. These will contain the least amount of saturated fats and also the most protein, vitamins, and minerals. Some fat is necessary to help the meat from drying out and provide better flavor. Although fat may be beneficial for cooking, it is important to try and skip unnecessary fats as much as possible.

One ounce of steak contains 55 calories, 3.3g of fat (1.2 saturated), 18mg of cholesterol, and 6g of protein. When compared to chicken or turkey, the protein levels aren't as high, but sometimes it's worth just having a grilled steak. After all, steak does contain creatine, which is essential for muscle growth. In comparison, poultry meats like chicken and turkey contain very little, if any, creatine.

If you are looking for the leanest cuts of steak, look for "loin" or "round" in the cut's name. If you don't care about the fat content, go for a Rib-eye. The Rib-eye steak has a marbled appearance that is said to have the best flavor of all cuts. This marbled appearance is due to the fat content.

The absolute best cuts of beef are bought through butchers. Buying half or a whole cow at one time through a private cattle farm is a great way to select your favorite cuts and have plenty of meat for later use.

Healthiest cuts of steak
Beef Eye Round Steak
Beef Top Round Steak
Beef Top Sirloin Steak
Beef Top Loin Strip Steak
Flank Steak
Fattiest cuts of steak
Rib-eye
New York
Strip Skirt Steak
Porterhouse / T-Bone

Pork

Pork is known as the other "white meat," but it is technically classified as a red meat. Pork is a fattier meat, so consuming the leaner portions is highly recommended. These are the tenderloins, loin chops, and loin roasts.

Pork contains 23g grams of protein and 12g of fat per every 3 ounces served (pork loin). Of the 12g of fat, 4.4g are saturated fat, which is not beneficial to overall cardiovascular health. Bacon typically contains 1g of fat per 1g of protein. When considering your food relationship, pork is something good to introduce once or twice a month, but it should not be a primary building block of your food relationship.

Pork is widely known as being an "unclean" meat; however, this typically stems from the religions of Judaism and Islam. Both Judaism and Islam prohibit the consumption of pork due to its uncleanliness and impurities (as outlined in the Torah for Judaism and the Quran for Islam). Although pigs and hogs do bathe in their own slop and are typically subjected to antibiotic treatments, outside of religious considerations the primary deterrent to consumption is the higher fat and cholesterol content.

Pork is also known to contain many worms and other bacteria that are harmful if not properly cooked. It is essential to get the internal temperature to at least 145° Fahrenheit (62.8° Celsius), and do not buy from any obscure or untrustworthy stores and restaurants. Try to also stay away from pork when traveling outside of the country, as cooking practices may be less regulated—primarily in South American countries.

Fish and Seafood

Fish is a power protein that should be included in your diet more often. They are plentiful in healthy fats (HDL) and oils, which most Americans lack the proper amount of in their diets. **Fish contain plenty of quality protein and healthy fats, and they are low in calories, contain vitamin B, vitamin D, and many other important minerals**. The American Heart Association even recommends eating fish twice a week to reap the benefits.

Fish comes in a variety of forms: fresh, frozen, and canned. So, which should you buy? There are some debates out there on which is best for you, but the primary considerations should be based on your needs, taste, and budget.

If you are looking for a quick snack or small meal, tuna and other canned fish is your absolute best option. If you are feeding more people, need larger portion sizes, or are looking for something that is more appealing in appearance and taste, fresh is the way to go. In comparison, frozen fish tends to lack flavor, but it is convenient for

Fish High In Healthy Fats
Salmon
Mackerel
Herring
Lake Trout
Sardines
Albacore Tuna

Healthiest Common Fish
Albacore Tuna
Salmon
Sardines
Rainbow Trout
Bluefin Tuna

Fish to Avoid
(Higher in mercury)
Shark
Swordfish
Tilefish
Salmon
Orange Roughy

a healthy meal. Many companies even individually seal the fish fillets to prevent freezer burn and allow for ease of use.

Buying fish can be a difficult process, especially if you are trying to buy quality fish. So what makes for quality fish? Two factors determine quality: where the fish comes from and how it was caught. If the fish is imported, there are typically fewer regulations and other unknown variables that may taint the quality of the product. This is why it is important to buy fish that is either wild caught, locally caught, or farmed in the United States. Catching your own fish or buying fish that is caught by hook and line, handline, or troll are the best options for ultra-lean and clean fish protein.

Confused that salmon is listed in both the categories of "Fish to Avoid" and the "Healthiest Common Fish"? If salmon is raised in a confined space like a fish farm, it is exposed to many chemicals that are not found in wild salmon. Always go with wild caught salmon.

Seafood (Shellfish)

Shellfish is another option when choosing seafood, including clams, oysters, mussels, shrimp, scallops, crab, and lobster. When thinking about your food relationship, shellfish is something that should only be occasionally considered—such as for special occasions like an anniversary or celebratory dinner.

My mother always reminded me "to stay away from anything that crawls on the ocean floor," and it always made me wonder why. Here's why: Apart from many shellfish being bottom-feeders, the meat in shellfish is typically higher in unhealthy cholesterol (LDL), higher in sodium, and often has a higher probability of containing unhealthy toxins. Shellfish allergies and post-ingestion sickness are also common, and this is one of the reasons why.

Recommend Shellfish Picks (in moderation)
Crab
Shrimp
Mussels
Scallops
Abalone
Oysters
Lobster
Squid

If you have high cholesterol, stay away from regular consumption of shrimp since they are higher in unhealthy cholesterol. An overall diet of less than 10 oz. of shellfish per week is a good rule of thumb to help prevent an excess intake of unhealthy cholesterol and toxins. But, next time you need a substitute for something other than chicken, beef or turkey, swap it up with some mussels or crab.

Meal preparation and purchasing is perhaps the most important part of eating shellfish. Shellfish should be cleaned thoroughly, bought from trusted sources, cooked properly, and stored appropriately.
If any of these links in the chain are broken, the potential for foodborne illness increases greatly.

When buying shellfish, one of the most important things to consider is how you are going to cook it. The cooking methods and sauces used determine how beneficial or detrimental it will be to your food relationship. You can bake, broil, deep fry, grill, steam, and boil your favorite shellfish meals. Just keep in mind that many of the healthy benefits that are synonymous with shellfish fade away when you fry them or add butter and other various sauces.

Shellfish is known to contain moderate levels of protein and the consumption of crab, clams mussels and oysters may actually help to lower unhealthy cholesterol levels.

Fruits and Vegetables

Fruits and vegetables are great additions to any diet. If you need to spice things up, fruits and vegetables are the answer. They add more vitamins and minerals to your diet and act as a great source of dietary fiber. Vegetables with protein also provide that protein with absolutely zero cholesterol. What is awesome about fruits and veggies is that they can be prepared in so many different ways. Vegetables can add texture and color to any meal and provide a healthy snack throughout the day.

When you are trying to piece together a meal, vegetables should be your secondary pick, right behind your protein. They will give you the vitamins and other nutrients that your protein doesn't provide, and they add color to your plate. Combining the right vegetables with your protein makes meals much more enjoyable.

Next time you are in the store, trying to figure out which fruits or vegetables to purchase, consider preference and taste. Buying foods that you like will help you eat more of them, so stick to the ones you like first and slowly branch out as you try more recipes.

Fresh vs Frozen, and Canned

Fresh vegetables are always your best option, but sometimes they may not be the most convenient or cost efficient. Surprisingly, canned and frozen vegetables are some of the freshest vegetables you can purchase. They go through the necessary preservation and decontamination processes, and they are sealed immediately after being picked. The preservation process (pasteurization, etc.) allows for more convenient storage and accessibility over time, which fresh vegetables cannot match. The taste may not be as extravagant, but it is pretty close. The frozen and canned options also help in a last minute bind when preparing a meal or needing a quick snack.

Canned and packaged options aren't a perfect alternative though. Keep in mind that many of these fruits and vegetables contain more sugar and sodium than their frozen counterparts. The sodium and sugar help to increase their shelf lives and maintain flavor. **Be observant when purchasing fruit and vegetables that are not on the perimeter of the store.**

Fruit cups are a perfect example of a sugar bomb in disguise, often containing 16-20+ grams of sugar per cup. Another great example of disaster in disguise are frozen vegetable dinners. Frozen vegetable dinners—even the "healthy" options—are

Fruits and vegetables can be found throughout the store, but not all of them have labels detailing whether they are low in sugar or salt. Check the ingredients. Just because food has fruits and vegetables in it does not mean it is healthy. Consider a single can of Campbell's Tomato Soup. One serving contains 480mg of sodium, 20g carbohydrates, and 12g of sugar. There are 2.5 servings per can, totaling 1200 mg of sodium. An average adult can typically eat one or two cans, but considering we should only take in about 1,000 mg of sodium per day, a single can of Campbell's soup equates to over an entire day's worth of salt!

packed full of sodium and other preservatives to avoid. **Look for "lower sodium," "no sugar added," or "no sodium added" when purchasing canned vegetables.** Adding tasty spices during preparation will offset the flavor differences. Whatever your choices may be, pick a variety of fruits and vegetables that are both colorful and can be added to a variety of dishes. Good examples are peppers, onions, tomatoes, spinach, and avocado.

If up to this point in your life, you have simply hated eating fruits and vegetables, it's probably because you've been preparing them wrong. Vegetables in particular can be cooked in a multitude of ways, accommodating to even the pickiest taste buds. Don't let those old memories of bland boiled vegetables ruin your relationship now.

GMO vs Organic Fruits and Vegetables

Many people gauge the health of their food relationship simply on how much "organic" produce they buy, but this is not an entirely accurate measurement, as there is much more to healthy food than just a label or sign. While in school for my horticultural degree, there were several heated debates in the classroom on the topic of organic produce. The class was divided, until the professor explained the real difference between organic and GMO produce.

There is so much controversy concerning organic and regular GMO produce (GMO, "Genetically Modified Organism" or GE, "Genetically Engineered"). While GMOs have been made to sound bad, a genetically modified organism can simply be cross-pollinating two different species. Many GMOs are created to help make produce that is disease, drought, and pest resistant. This increases the amount of food that can be produced and consumed. There have not been any detrimental results from the produce itself or on the farmland where they are cultivated. GMOs also save you tons of money.

Consider tomatoes or other vegetables you have grown in your own garden. They sometimes look funny even though they taste delicious, but in order to sell fruit and vegetables in an open market, your harvest would need to look nearly perfect—just think about how picky you are when selecting the best produce at the grocery store (size, shape, and color matter). If the organic produce market were to use absolutely no assistance of chemicals to grow their products, their yield for an open market would be extremely low. This would cause produce to be triple the current price. To increase their revenues and product yield, the organic products utilize USDA-approved pesticides and fertilizers. The best thing going for the organic market is that it is slightly more regulated than that of certain GMO crops; however, this does not mean they are healthier for you. Ironically, GMOs and organic crops share virtually identical nutrition numbers.

Also, despite many of the USDA regulations, most "organic" produce is shipped in from overseas, where there is little to no regulation for chemicals, treatment, or cultivating practices. Keep this in mind next time you buy organic that is not from local farms.

So what's the best option? **Buy local.** Although there may not be any "regulations" for local farmers, you have a better chance of buying completely natural vegetables that haven't undergone the shipping processes and regular chemical treatments—and you can forget worrying about buying products that are made in other countries. You may come across the occasional farmer who used a little Miracle Gro on their plants and nitrogen in their soil, which is no big deal.

If you are still skeptical about GMOs, there are two lists that are helpful when buying produce. They are the "dirty dozen" and "clean fifteen." When it comes down to it, fruits and vegetables with softer skins tend to be eaten by insects more, which means increased pesticide applications. **The clean fifteen use fewer chemicals (thicker skins) while the dirty dozen typically use more (thinner skins).** Also, buying produce while it is in season helps reduce cost and improve the quality of the product.

Dirty Dozen	Clean Fifteen
Apples	Asparagus
Blueberries	Avocado
Celery	Cabbage
Cucumbers	Cantaloupe
Grapes	Eggplant
Lettuce	Grapefruit
Nectarines	Honeydew Melon
Peaches	Kiwi
Potatoes	Mangos
Spinach	Onions
Strawberries	Pineapple
Sweet bell peppers	Sweet Corn
	Sweet Peas
	Sweet Potato
	Watermelon

Breads and Whole Grains

Breads and whole grains are great additions to nearly any meal. They provide a myriad of health benefits, give you a boost of energy, and are loaded with nutrients, vitamins, and minerals. Whole grains are known to include protein, fiber, vitamins B and E, and trace minerals such as iron, zinc, and magnesium.

If you are not sure which breads are the healthiest options, check the amount of fiber on the back—the higher the fiber, the better. Higher fiber typically accounts for a less refined product. Keep in mind that the calories in each slice are also dependent upon the size, bread type, slice thickness, sugar added, and salt content.

Whole grains have even been proven to reduce the risk of heart disease, diabetes and cancer. White breads, bleached flours, and any "refined" or "white" grains typically go through more processing. If it doesn't say "whole wheat" or "whole grain," it is more refined and less healthy. If the packaging states "100%," then all of the grain is whole wheat or whole grain, and these are your healthiest options.

When you walk through the store aisles, bread and wheat products made with bread-like substance (carbohydrates, such as crackers, snacks, cereals, and pastas) are everywhere. Remember the five rules when considering carbs. As you creep into the inner aisles, the expiration dates are much longer, which should raise a flag of caution. Try to go with the 100% whole-wheat and whole grain crackers, pastas, and cereals. They are typically about the same price as their unhealthy counterpart and don't taste too much different.

There are some snacks in the aisles like crackers and chips that you may feel you just have to have. Two snacks I personally

"If you can't moderate, eliminate."

love are Goldfish crackers and Wheat Thins. I know if I don't portion out the little fish or crackers, I can easily eat almost an entire box in one sitting. This is the dark side of snacks and quick 'n easy bread products. **They are addictive!** The whole wheat healthier options of both Wheat Thins and Goldfish still contain a high amount of sodium and carbohydrates, which when eaten en-masse will sabotage even the cleanest of diets. **That's what is so crazy about boxed and instant foods—their sodium and fat contents are literally addictive.** Our bodies crave those two things and get a "high" from eating them. So, enjoy your favorite carb snacks *in moderation*, and know that your relationship with food is more important than one little "cheat," which could ruin your nutrition goals.

Ask yourself these questions when you are going down the store aisles:
1. Is the bread or grain product 100% Whole Wheat, Whole Wheat or Whole Grain?
2. What is the expiration date? Fresh bread(s) and whole grain products should have relatively short expiration dates (1-2 weeks).
3. Where is it located in the store?
4. Is it made from the bakery or highly packaged in individualized wrappers? The less packaging the better.

Bread has been known to ruin many fantastic food relationships, spinning even a healthy relationship into one of addiction. Let's consider one piece of bread. One piece of bread can be anywhere from 60-150+ calories per slice, depending on the type of bread and thickness of the slice. When eating a sandwich, the median calorie count of 100 calories per slice

Recommended Breads and Whole Grains
100% Whole Wheat Bread, Flour, Crackers, etc.
100% Whole Grain Bread
Brown Rice
Millet
Quinoa
Sorghum
Triticale
Whole Grain Barley
Whole Grain Corn
Whole Wheat Couscous
Whole Wheat Oatmeal / Oats / Steel Cut
Wild Rice

equals 200 calories per sandwich. If you decide to have a second sandwich, the bread alone will account for approximately 400 calories in that single meal, or 1/5 of the typical 2,000 calorie a day intake. This doesn't even account for the non-sliced breads, such as loaves and buns that have much higher calorie counts. Just think about how much bread you can scarf down at a restaurant before you even eat the main meal. Bottom line, bread has many great nutritional aspects, but it unfortunately packs plenty of calories with little satiety.

Nutrition for Top Five Recommended Breads

1. 100% Whole Wheat Bread (Sara Lee Classic)

Calories	Total Fat	Carbs	Protein	Sugar	Cholesterol	Sodium	Fiber
60	1g	12g	3g	1g	0 mg	120 mg	2g

2. Ezekiel 4:9 Bread

Calories	Total Fat	Carbs	Protein	Sugar	Cholesterol	Sodium	Fiber
80	5g	14g	4g	0g	0 mg	80 mg	3g

3. Flaxseed Bread (Healthy Life)

Calories	Total Fat	Carbs	Protein	Sugar	Cholesterol	Sodium	Fiber
90	.5g	8g	4g	3g	0 mg	80 mg	2g

4. Oat Bread (Pepperidge Farm Whole Grain Oatmeal Bread)

Calories	Total Fat	Carbs	Protein	Sugar	Cholesterol	Sodium	Fiber
101	.5g	21g	5g	4g	0 mg	125 mg	3g

5. Rye Bread (Pepperidge Farm Dell Swirl – Rye & Pumpernickel)

Calories	Total Fat	Carbs	Protein	Sugar	Cholesterol	Sodium	Fiber
80	1g	14g	3g	1g	0 mg	200 mg	1g

Desserts and Sweets

Ah, sweets. They are typically the staple to end any night, especially when you eat out at a restaurant. Perhaps the craziest part about sweets is how many calories are crammed into such a small amount. Nearly all desserts are caloric dense and can unravel your food relationship in no time. Some of the "healthier" desserts, containing fruit or labeled low fat, can even sabotage your weight loss goals. So, how do you still eat dessert and not overdo it? By keeping your goals in mind and not letting impulse decisions destroy your food relationship.

Good alternatives to regular "desserts" or sweets (in moderation)
Fruit
Cacao Chocolate (60-85%)
Cocoa Chocolate (Dark)
Low Fat / No Sugar ice cream
Dark chocolate covered almonds
Low fat frozen yogurt
Semi-sweet chocolate morsels
Italian Ice (check nutrition label)
One small scoop of ice cream (vanilla or chocolate) with fresh fruit

Dessert Challenge

Because dessert can ruin some of the best diets, it is a good idea to write down your triggers. Knowing what triggers your impulses is extremely important when trying to stay on the narrow nutritional path. At first it may be difficult, but that's because sugar is highly addictive. Keep your long-term goals in mind and success will shortly follow.

Should I eliminate dessert from my diet? Why?

How much dessert should I buy? Why?

What is considered a sweet or dessert? First thoughts?

What are your sweet cravings? What are your dessert vices?

Due to the addictive nature of dessert and sugary treats, it is often best to avoid them altogether. This is especially true if you have a habit of overeating. If there is no temptation present, you cannot falter. If you have enough self-control to limit your sweets intake, then the most difficult decision will be deciding which *one* to purchase.

Cravings for sweets are normal—that's why it's not always best to completely abstain from sweets unless you are a person who can't stop eating them once you start. **Sweets are detrimental to your diet, but it is possible to eat them without gaining weight.** When eating sweets, go for healthier options and smaller portions in the earlier hours of the afternoon. If you do have a sweet tooth, fruits are made up of natural sugars that can sometimes crush the desire without all the unnecessary calories.

Keep in mind that sweets don't have to be just cake, chocolate, candies, cookies, or ice cream. They can be disguised as carbonated beverages and juices. Many sodas, juices, and sports drinks are absolutely loaded with sugar. Companies increase the sugar content to make the drinks tastier and more appealing to all age groups. Next time you are looking to buy something other than milk, water, tea, or coffee, check the sugar content. You may be surprised just how much those beverages are destroying your diet.

One of the best ways to conquer that sweet tooth is to make sure you eat plenty of food during your meals. Don't save room for dessert because it takes up more room in your calorie plan that you would like to even know. The best way to forgo these button-busters is to just forget about them when you go shopping.

Beverages

Apart from desserts, liquid calories are the fastest food relationship destroyers. With this in mind, minimize your variety of drinks when shopping. The more you buy, the higher the chance of buying a calorie bomb. Nearly all sodas and carbonated beverages contain preservatives, artificial sweeteners, sugar, and sodium. Try to minimize or eliminate soda—that includes "diet" versions—and limit your juice and sweet tea to one or two glasses a day. Even though juices are tastier and healthier than soda, they are still loaded with sugar and can be just as detrimental.

Best to worst beverages
Water
Tea & Coffee
Milk
Juices
Soda / Carbonated
Beverages
Alcohol

Water

When it comes to your body, water is one the most important aspects of your relationship. Despite the significance of water and how it helps the body, it is often one of the most neglected and forgotten about aspects of a healthy diet. Water helps you stay hydrated, flush out toxins, regulate body temperature, aid in weight loss, improve digestion, and overall make your body work more efficiently—just to name a few things. Water also contains absolutely no calories.

Recommended intake of water is about .5 oz per pound or 1.1 oz per kg. Rough approximations place the average intake

Buying a gallon jug or larger reusable container can help you keep track of just how much water you drink throughout the day.

for males at about ½-¾ a gallon per day and ½ gallon per day for females. With exercise or environmental exposures, such as heat and cold, increase your intake and replace lost water. If you are starting to get bored with water, add flavor with a lemon or lime slice, berries, oranges, mint leaves, or water additive like Crystal Light or Mio. Eating fruits and vegetables is also a great way to ingest water without even realizing it. Many fruits and vegetables are made primarily of water.

Recommended Daily Consumption of Water
1 Gallon = 128 oz / ¾ Gallon = 96 oz / ½ Gallon = 64 oz

Weight (lbs / kg)	Recommended Ounces
100 / 45.5	50
125 / 56.8	62.5
150 / 68.2	75
175 / 79.5	87.5
200 / 90.9	100
225 / 102.2	112.5
250 / 113.6	125
275 / 125	137.5
300 / 136.4	150

Tea and Coffee

Tea and coffee are fantastic additions to your everyday diet. It's what you put in tea and coffee that may ruin your relationship. Tea and coffee have virtually no calories after they are brewed (roughly 5 cal per cup). A cup of green tea, like coffee, can also be a nice little kick to a slow afternoon as it contains 30-75mg of caffeine per cup.

Tea is known to have many antioxidants, heart and weight loss benefits, and qualities to help lower cholesterol levels. When compared to coffee, a cup of tea is actually recommended over the cup of Joe. If you are going to drink tea, stick with the home-brewed teas and avoid the pre-packaged teas in plastic drink containers since they contain more sugar and preservatives. Opt for green tea, black tea, white tea, and herbal teas as they are your absolute healthiest options.

There's nothing quite like a cup of coffee in the morning. Just be careful what you put in your coffee. That is where the calories and cholesterol pile up. Apart from the additives, coffee is known to boost your energy, help burn fat, and has even been said to help prevent diabetes and heart disease. Just like tea, your healthiest option is home-brewed coffee. Stay away from the sugar-laden coffee like macchiato, frappuccino, cafe mochas, and lattes if you are planning to stay within your daily calorie limit. The recommended daily intake is only 2-4 cups of coffee and/or tea—and that's not venti sized.

Milk

Unless you are lactose intolerant, you should highly consider introducing milk into your regular diet. Milk is known to contain calcium, vitamin C, vitamin D, potassium, and magnesium. There are many other vitamins such as B12, B6, A, and riboflavin that are also found in small amounts in milk. Calcium and vitamins C & D help strengthen bones and teeth, while the other vitamins help regulate sleep, coagulate blood, improve mood, improve immune system function, decrease hypertension, and relieve muscle pain.

With all the varieties of milk on the market today, it may be difficult to determine which one is most beneficial for your diet. Listed below are some quick explanations of the most popular varieties of milk in the store today.

Whole Milk and Vitamin D Milk

Whole Milk and Vitamin D Milk provide a rich and creamy taste, but they contain higher levels of fat and more calories. Go for either of these milks if you are not as concerned with your calorie or fat intake. Milk lovers typically stick with whole milk and Vitamin D Milk, as they prefer the consistency and flavor. Keep in mind that liquid calories are easy to over consume, ruining your daily caloric intake goals.

2%, 1%, Skim, and Chocolate Milk

When comparing all three of these milks, fat content is the primary difference. 2% will have the most fat, followed by 1%, and then skim milk. If you are looking to have a similar consistency to that of whole milk and Vitamin D milk, go for 2%.

If you want a good mix between 2% and skim milk, 1% is your best option. If you are looking to drink milk but need to skip the calories, skim milk is your best option. Skim milk simply contains less fat than its counterparts, while still maintaining the vitamins and minerals. *Skim milk is the healthiest milk containing lactose.*

Chocolate milk is higher in calories, fat, sugar, and protein. This cocoa flavored milk variety is great to drink in small quantities or even as a post-workout drink, but try to stay away from regular consumption, as it is caloric dense.

Soy Milk, Almond Milk, and Coconut Milk

Soy, almond, and coconut milks are great alternatives to regular milk. They do not contain lactose, making them ideal for those who are lactose-intolerant. Almond and coconut milk are recommended for both men and women, whereas soy milk is more beneficial for women. Soy milk has been said to increase the estrogen levels in men and may be associated with other medical issues. If you are a man and wary of the possible side effects of soy milk, just go for almond milk.

Something else to keep in mind is the extended shelf lives of lactose-free milks. They are often found in the inner aisles of the grocery store, and their expiration dates can be significantly longer than those of their lactose containing counterparts.

Top Milk with Lactose
Skim Milk
1% Milk
2% Milk
Whole Milk
Vitamin D Milk
Chocolate Milk
Top Lactose-Free Milks
Almond Milk
Coconut Mil
Soy Milk

Remember, the longer the expiration date, the more preservatives.

If you don't feel like milk, don't forget the other dairy: cheese. Cheese is perceived as an essential part of many meals today. Unfortunately, cheese is extremely high in fat, sodium, and cholesterol—not to mention calories. The average amount of calories per slice of cheese is 60. This equates to a half-mile jog. If you are trying to watch what you eat, just check how much cheese you are consuming because you might be surprised.

Juices: Fruit and Vegetable

Juices were a staple in my family growing up, and that's a good thing. Fruit juices are popular for having many unique flavors and providing several essential vitamins and nutrients. Even though you can obtain key vitamins and nutrients, juice can also be very high in sugar content. So, if you don't want to offset the nutritional benefits with high amounts of sugar, purchase juices that have reduced sugar or no sugar added. Purchasing 100% all natural juice is also a great option, as it helps reduce the amount of preservatives and artificial sweeteners. Even juices from concentrate contain high amounts of sugar and preservatives.

Another type of popular juice on the market today is vegetable juice. Vegetable juices are great for boosting your immune system and

Top Juice Picks
V8 Vegetable Juice, Low Sodium
V8 100% Vegetable Juice
Orange Juice
Apple Juice
Pineapple Juice
Pomegranate Juice

helping you include more vitamins in your daily diet. Drinking vegetables is an easy way to introduce more vegetables to your daily diet without cooking or having long prep times. Canned vegetable drinks are low in sugar compared to fruit juices; however, the sodium content is much higher. Using a juicer is a great way to drink healthy vegetables throughout the day, either as a snack or meal replacement. Just keep in mind that because there is a lack of sugar in vegetables, they are slightly more difficult to drink and consume in mass quantity.

Overall, fruit and vegetable juices are a great addition to any diet if in moderation (1-2 cups per day). In the long run, consuming real fruits and vegetables in their entirety is the best option. Eating the entire fruit or vegetable gives you more vitamins and nutrients than you could receive from just drinking the juice.

Carbonated Beverages

Carbonated beverages are sold all over the world and are found in almost every household. However, despite the popularity of these fizzy drinks, they are some of the least healthy items you can consume. Carbonated drinks contain tons of sugar and are laced with artificial sweeteners and preservatives. Soda is a direct contributor to obesity and early-onset diabetes—two health plagues that are sweeping society today.

Soda is so caloric dense, that if you cut it out of your diet, you can expect to see the pounds start

If you do decide to have a fizzy drink, opt for the "Low Calorie," "Zero Sugar Added" or "No Caffeine" options.

to fall off. Cutting it out entirely is important, although it may be extremely difficult. Soda contains sugar and caffeine, which are both addictive substances. Cutting sugar and/or caffeine out may take some time, especially if they have been consumed in excess. The fight to reduce or eliminate the unhealthy carbonated beverages from your life will be worth it though, especially if you are looking to have a successful long-term relationship with food.

Many friends and clients of mine who have cut soda begin feeling better almost instantly. They are also excited to see the numbers drop on the scale.

There is really no "top pick" for carbonated beverages or sodas. Stay away from them if at all possible.
Carbonated Water (various flavors)
Ginger Ale
Sprite
Red Bull Total Zero

Alcohol

You may have a favorite beer or mixed drink, but that drink may be sabotaging your food relationship more than other things. Alcohol is one of the biggest reasons for weight gain because it consists almost entirely of empty calories, contains no nutrients, and is often consumed in great quantity.

You can drink easily 12-20+ beers over the weekend, but all those calories have to go somewhere—typically to your gut and butt. Let's take a light beer like a 12oz Bud Light for example.

Drink eight of those. You just racked up close to 900 calories. This does not even include special seasonal beers, rums, etc. that are even higher in calories. To burn off, that's about eight miles-worth of running. Three glasses of wine equates to three miles worth of running. Beware and be aware.

As for mixed drinks, they wreak more havoc than light beers. They are filled with sugar and packed with calories. You may have two or three mixed drinks, but that can equate to more than 1,000 calories in no time. Although a large percentage of the calories come from the alcohol, the remainder of the calories are from mixers like sodas.

Apart from the temporary therapeutic feelings you might get from drinking alcohol, alcohol is simply disastrous to your caloric needs for the day and provides little to no nutritional benefit of any kind.

So, if you are going to drink, drink smart. Don't start drinking if you know you can't stop. Alcohol is so easy to overconsume that it should be considered with extreme caution if you are trying to lose weight and become healthier. **Be smart when buying alcohol to keep your food relationship on track.**

Top Recommendations for Alcohol Choices (based on calories)

Wine

Wine makes the top of the list simply because red wines contain polyphenols (antioxidants that help fight free radicals in your body that may encourage the growth of cancer and other diseases). Wines are also typically consumed with meals and less likely to be overindulged on like beer or liquor.

Clear Liquors

Clear liquors are lighter on the calories than darker liquors. They are even lower on the calories when ordered neat (straight) or on the rocks (on ice). Drinking straight liquor can take some adjustment time, but it is more likely to be sipped slower than beer, mixed drinks, or wine coolers. The higher the proof (the measure of alcohol content), the higher alcohol and calorie content. If you add soda or juice, you shoot the calories through the roof.

Light Beers

Light beer comes in last mostly because they are typically consumed in large quantities. If you can get away with drinking one light beer or maybe two, that's great but not typical, especially during big parties or events. Beer is full of empty calories and carbs that are not beneficial to your health. When you want to drink it, stick to the lower calorie choices to keep your food relationship on track, even during those "cheat meals." Cider beers, IPAs, microbrews, stouts, and lagers are not good alternatives unless you can drink only one or two, as they often double or triple the calories of light beer.

Wine Calories

Wine Types	Calories Per Glass (5 oz)	Calories Per Bottle
Reds: Cabernet Sauvignon, Merlot, Pinot Noir, Syrah, Malbec, Zinfandel	125	650
Whites: Chardonnay, Sauvignon Blanc, Pinot Gris (Grigio), Riesling, Moscato	120	625

Liquor Calories

Alcohol Type	Proof	Ounces	Calories
Vodka	80	1	64
		1.5 (shot)	97
Tequila	80	1	64
		1.5 (shot)	97
Rum / Whiskey	86	1	70
		1.5 (shot)	105
Gin	90	1	73
		1.5 (shot)	110

Light Beer Calories

Light Beers	Calories Per 12 Ounces
Bud Select	55
Miller MGD 64	64
Becks Premier Light	64
Amstel Light	95
Busch Light	95
Yuengling Light Lager	95
Natural Light	95
Corona Light	99
Coors Light	102
Bud Light	110

Going Steady Summary

With tens of thousands of options in the store, you are now ready to navigate the aisles and take your relationship with food to the next level. You are now ready to go steady and get serious about healthy food in a way that will not only change your life but also your loved ones'.

Like any serious relationship, you learn new things about yourself and your loved one as time progresses—it is no different with food. You will find where the healthy food is stashed away in your favorite store, figure out which foods compliment your taste buds, and even which healthy foods to default to in times of desperation.

Let's put all this effort to use and finish up with a question section to see how your opinions or views of food have changed.

Are You Ready to Go Steady?

Do you think your original shopping list will still stand up the rigors of healthy eating? Let's find out.

What surprised you the most throughout this section? Why?

Based on your previous shopping list, what are some foods that you can now substitute for the less-healthy versions? (Examples: Turkey instead of Beef)

Which foods have you added to your list? Subtracted?

Which foods are you going to stay away from now?

Food is awesome, so let's keep it that way. With a proper balance of protein, fruits, vegetables, complex carbohydrates, and even some sweets or occasional alcohol, you can enjoy countless varieties of awesome food dates.

Don't forget that **your goals of weight loss or weight gain _are_ possible with patience and perseverance.** Keeping your goals in mind will increase your chances of long-term success. Any foods or drinks that can hinder these goals are best to be removed from your cabinets and diet altogether. Eliminating the unhealthy temptations will prepare you for victory, day-in and day-out.

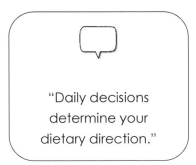

"Daily decisions
determine your
dietary direction."

PART THREE:
Understanding the Science

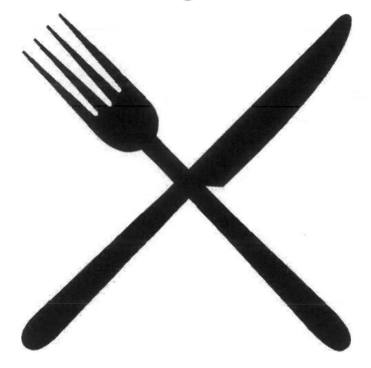

Understanding the Love of Food: The Nutritional Science of the Simple and Healthy Food Relationship

For some, science is boring, but when it comes to explaining your food relationship, science is a bit more interesting. After all, science has everything to do with food. Science shows you which foods are healthy for you, why they are healthy, and their direct impact on your body. Everything you know about your body, what foods you put in it, and what those foods do it is science. This is why it is important to now learn "what" and "why" certain foods are good or bad for you.

Although this section is an oversimplified version of food science, it will help to point you in the right direction when you need a quick reference or explanation. You won't need to worry about complex equations or the adverse chemical reactions that occur during the cooking process, only the basics.

Time to get nerdy. Take notes because some of these quick facts will help you catalyze your food relationship faster than you think.

Love = Calories

Food is made up of calories, and if you want to have a healthy diet, you need to know what they are. So before venturing any further into the nutritional science, let's talk about the little thing called a calorie. **Simply put, a calorie is a measurement of energy.**

> One calorie = Increases the temperature of one gram of water, 1 degree Celsius
> One Calorie (kcal) = Increases the temperature of one kilogram of water, 1 degree Celsius

For the sake of food, it is proper to refer to calories as **kcal (kilocalories)** or **C**alories. If the "C" is capitalized, then you are talking about a kilocalorie, and not the smaller measurement of energy, calorie. However, for this book, we will refer to Calories or kcal simply as "calories." Next time you see a capitalized "C" or "kcal," you will know exactly what it means.

Believe it or not, certain foods are more flammable than others. This relates directly to their calories. If you are sitting around the campfire making s'mores, what is the most common food to go up in flames? You got it, marshmallows. One of the reasons is due to its caloric density, or the potential energy it contains (made of sugar and gelatin). Obviously you aren't going to be putting your graham cracker over the fire, but even if you did right next to the marshmallow, the graham cracker would take longer to catch on fire due to the decreased caloric density when compared to the marshmallow.

This can be true for vegetables and other foods that are not as caloric dense and more natural. Natural foods (vegetables and meat) take much longer to burn, and therefore they are more beneficial to the inner workings and operations of your body. The longer something takes to burn, the better your body can utilize it for energy.

Simple food science says to stick with the foods that don't catch on fire as easily. Everything will burn eventually, but you want to introduce foods to your body that are substantive and of quality. **Most foods that are high in calories are low quality foods: junk foods, fats, and processed foods.** This is true even amongst healthier foods, where some options are better than others. Consider meats that are higher in fat, such as beef and pork, which

"Eat clean, for clean fuel burns more efficiently."

have more of a tendency to flare up on the grill compared to chicken. Why? It's due to the fat content. Fat equals high calories, which means it burns faster and hotter (a calorimeter is utilized to measure this process).

If you take in more calories (potential energy) than your body needs, then you will begin to store them as fat, creating a reserve of energy as a natural means of survival. Although the extra storage of energy may seem like a good idea in times of need, we are not cavemen, and very few people in society go on extended journeys where extra fat would be beneficial. Bottom line, if you take in too many calories, you will gain weight.

Understanding what a calorie (kcal) is and how it can affect your eating habits is key to improving your food relationship. The more you know about the food you are eating, the better your relationship will be. Sound familiar?

Love Comes in All Sizes: Micro's and Macro's

Relationships are intricate in nature, undergoing both major and minor events to remain strong over time and survive various trials. When it comes to food, our major events will be equated with macronutrients or "macro's." The minor events, still completely necessary for overall health, are known as micronutrients or "micro's."

You need both macro and micronutrients in your diet to meet all of your body's demands. Our bodies require a variety of nutrients, both big and small, from many different foods to operate effectively. Also, our bodies are subjected to a variety of challenges, which demand big and small nutrients to be victorious. These challenges may be viewed as our basic immune system, physical movement, maintenance, and really anything that deals with the body.

Another way to think about micro and macronutrients is equating them with building blocks. Macronutrients are the larger building blocks, as they constitute for the bulk of the food material and calories in food. Micronutrients act as the mortar holding the blocks together. They are not measured in calories, but rather in percentages, milligrams, or other small units of measurement. Both are equally important. If you lack either one, the body will be weaker and subject to various threats. A diet that is well-balanced and full of quality foods will provide an ample supply of building blocks and mortar to operate and strengthen the body efficiently.

Many people like to base their diets around how many macronutrients and micronutrients they are consuming. They are essentially measuring the amount of building blocks necessary to perform regular daily functions and aid the body when it may need more (for exercise, etc.).

Micronutrients

Micronutrients, a.k.a. vitamins and minerals, are key components of a well-balanced diet. They act as the mortar for the body, allowing everything to function properly in conjunction with the macronutrients. Some of the primary vitamins are calcium, chloride, sodium, magnesium, phosphorus, and potassium, with trace elements being that of iron and zinc. Eating a healthy diet will supply your body with plenty of vitamins and minerals.

If there are imbalances with certain vitamins, physical symptoms will occur as a result. Signs and symptoms vary depending on which vitamins or minerals the body is deficient. One of the best ways you can make sure you are not deficient in necessary vitamins or minerals is to take a multivitamin.

Micronutrients: The Multivitamin

Multivitamins can aid many diets; however, they are not always necessary. If you eat a well-rounded diet with plenty of fruits, vegetables, whole grains, and lean meats, it is unlikely that you need to take a multivitamin or have any nutritional deficiencies. Healthy foods are packed with tons of vitamins and minerals.

Doctors will typically prescribe multivitamins or similar supplements when there are notable deficits in blood labs, foreseeable body changes, such as pregnancy, or a condition that cannot be corrected with proper diet and exercise. The best way to determine this is with a visit to your doctor and nutritionist.

When it comes to overall nutritional intake and multivitamins, alternative eating styles, such as vegetarianism and veganism, are typically a topic of discussion. Vegetarians and vegans often eat plenty of essential vitamins and nutrients in their diets, as their intake of fruits and vegetables is higher than most. One might assume that they would not need any additional supplementation in the form of a multivitamin. However, this is not always true as there are many vitamins and minerals missing from a purely plant-base diet.

Although a multivitamin may not be needed for vegetarians or vegans, more attention should be addressed to other vitamins and minerals that their diets often lack. Certain vitamins, such vitamins B_{12}, vitamin D, calcium, iron, and zinc, must often be added by supplementation or vitamin-enriched foods, as they are not as prevalent or are completely absent from an animal-free diet. A good example is B_{12}, as it is only found in certain meats.

Next time you are thinking about taking a multivitamin, ask yourself, "am I eating a well-balanced diet, full of fruits, vegetables, and lean proteins?" If not, a multivitamin may be good for you.

Top Vitamin Picks
Vitamin B12 / B6
Vitamin D
Calcium
Iron
Vitamin C
Folic Acid
Fish Oil

Vitamins: Where to Find Them and What They Do

Vitamin / Mineral	Function	Foods Containing
Calcium	Bone and Teeth Health, Heart and Nerve Health	Milk, Kale, Sardines, Yogurt, Cheese, Bok Choy, Almonds
Cobalamin (B12)	Nervous System Health	Cooked Clams, Beef Liver, Fish, Crab, Fortified Foods
Fish Oil / Omega 3's	Reduce Triglycerides, Improves Heart and Cardiovascular Health	Fish, Flaxseed Oil, Chia Seeds, Oysters, Soybeans, Spinach
Folic Acid	Red Blood Cell Production	Lentils, Dried Beans, Avocado, Broccoli, Spinach, Citrus fruits, Organ Meats
Iron	Helps transport Oxygen	Liver, Oysters, Clams, Chickpeas, Fortified Cereals, Soybeans, Chicken, Turkey, Fish, Red meats, Organ Meats
Niacin (B3)	Metabolism, Digestive and	Fish, Chicken, Turkey, Pork, Peanuts, Mushrooms, Potatoes,

	Nervous System Health	Eggs, Enriched Cereals
Potassium	Aids in Nervous System Function and Muscle Contraction	Avocado, Banana, Sweet Potato, Spinach, Acorn Squash, Black Beans, Lean Meats
Pyrodoxin (B6)	Metabolism, Red Blood Cell Production	Sunflower Seeds, Pistachios, Tuna, Turkey, Chicken, Avocados, Dried Beans
Riboflavin (B2)	Metabolism, Skin and Eye Health	Cheese, Almonds, Beef, Lamb, Eggs, Fish, Whole Grains, Organ Meats
Thiamine (B1)	Metabolism and Nerve Function	Fish, Pork, Beef, Seeds, Nuts, Bread, Green Peas, Whole Grains, Liver
Vitamin A (Beta-Carotene)	Vision, Skin, Bone and Tooth growth, Immune System	Carrots, Sweet Potatoes, Squash, Spinach, Kale, Broccoli, Dairy Products
Vitamin C - Ascorbic Acid	Protein Metabolism, Immune System, Iron Absorption	Peppers, Kale, Kiwi, Broccoli, Berries, Citrus Fruits

Vitamin D	Absorption of Calcium and Maintain Strong Bones	Sunlight (non-food), Cod Liver Oil, Fish, Milk, Eggs, Mushrooms
Vitamin E	Antioxidant, Protects Cells	Spinach, Almonds, Sunflower Seeds, Avocados, Fish, Squash, Spinach

Macronutrients

Macronutrients are the "large" molecules known as carbohydrates, proteins, and fats. These molecules are the building blocks that the body utilizes for energy, maintenance, and every other essential body function. "Counting macro's" is a common term utilized when someone is trying to eat a specific amount of carbohydrates, protein, and fat. Carbohydrates, proteins, and fat are all necessary for the body to operate as it should. They should be consumed every day and in sufficient amounts. Refer to calorie counting for your daily intake percentages.

Macronutrients - Based on a 2,000 Calorie/Day Diet

Macronutrient	Energy Per Gram	Recommended %	With Exercise %
Carbohydrates	4 kcal / g	55-65	55-70
Protein	4 kcal / g	15-35	20-40
Fat	9 kcal / g	10-15	20-40

The Skinny on Fat

Eating fat is essential for any healthy diet and healthy food relationship. Eating the right kinds of fat and the right amount is the balancing act. It is very easy to consume too many unhealthy fats, as they make up many of the foods in our grocery stores today.

Fat contains a whopping **9 kcal per gram,** and it is recommended not to let fats count for more than **25-30% of your dietary intake**. Due to fat's caloric density, it is easy to consume too many calories in a single sitting. There are many great health benefits of fat, but again, eating the right kind is the key. There are four types of fat: saturated fat, unsaturated fat, trans fat, and triglycerides. Stick with unsaturated fats, limit saturated fats, and stay away from trans fats.

If you are eating a healthy diet with lean meats and plenty of fiber, you shouldn't stress too much over your daily fat intake. Also, instead of worrying about how many grams of fat per pound/kg you should be eating, ask the question "what percentage of my daily intake should fat be?" Rather than trying to critique the grams per day, stick to your percentages, only worrying about kinds of fat and the overall impact on your diet.

"Sats make me fat, unsats make me un-fat, trans don't make future plans."

Quick Breakdowns for a 2,000 kcal Diet

Daily % Fat Intake	Kcal per Day of Fat	Grams of Fat per Day
10	200	22
20	400	44
25	500	55
30	600	66

Saturated Fat

Saturated fats are typically solid at room temperature. Examples of saturated fat are **butter, cheese, margarine, and the fat that surrounds animal meats**. Leaner cuts of meat are recommended for consumption as they contain less saturated fat, decreasing your risk of heart disease. Greater intake of saturated fats typically leads to increased cholesterol levels and high blood pressure.

The American Heart Association recommends that only 5-6% of your daily diet consist of saturated fats. On a 2,000 kcal diet with 25% fat intake, 5% of saturated fat constitutes for around 100 kcal or 11g.

Trans Fat

Trans fats are artificial or manufactured fats that are added to preserve foods for abnormal amounts of time, as well as alter taste and texture. Foods with trans fat typically have long shelf lives, contain partially hydrogenated vegetable oils, and may be found in foods like cookies, cakes, pie crusts, frozen pizzas, stick margarines, fried foods, and doughnuts. It is recommended to consume less than 1% of trans fat per day. It is directly linked with increased Low Density Lipoprotein (LDL) cholesterol levels and diabetes. You want your LDL levels to be as low as possible, and trans fats do not help.

Unsaturated Fat

Unsaturated fats or "oils" are often liquid at room temperatures and are typically derived from plant sources or fish. **Examples of unsaturated fats are salad dressings, the oil surrounding tuna, and cooking oils**. Two branches of unsaturated fats are polyunsaturated fats and monounsaturated fats.

Polyunsaturated and monounsaturated fats are known to lower bad (LDL) cholesterol, while maintaining good High Density Lipoprotein (HDL) cholesterol levels. They also contain vitamin E and help cell function throughout the body. The main sources of polyunsaturated and monounsaturated fats are canola oil, olive oil, corn oil, cereal oil, safflower oil, and sunflower oil. Don't worry too much about the difference between mono and polyunsaturated fats, as it is moderately insignificant when it comes to your overall eating habits. On the molecular level, monounsaturated and polyunsaturated fats have different bonds, but they still maintain similar health benefits and are both liquid at room temperature.

Eat unsaturated fats, consume fewer saturated fats, and STAY AWAY from trans fats.

Top Fat Picks
Salmon
Mackerel
Almonds
Avocado
Eggs
Nuts
Seeds
Olive Oil

What is Cholesterol?

Cholesterol is a waxy substance that is similar to fat. It is found throughout our bodies and helps regulate hormones, aid in cell function, and assist in many other bodily functions. Just like with fat, having the right kinds and right amounts of cholesterol in the body is the key. This is where a proper diet is important again.

The more healthy fats consumed, the better LDL (Low Density Lipoprotein), HDL (High Density Lipoprotein), and triglyceride levels will be. Cholesterol and triglyceride levels are important blood markers to help determine the prevalence of heart disease, high blood pressure, and stroke.

If you or a loved one has high cholesterol levels, there are a couple things outside of regularly taking your prescribed medicines that you can do to help. Consuming foods that have healthy fats reduces the chance of plaque buildup and provides your body with energy that it can use. Regular exercise is also one of the best habits you can start for lowering unhealthy cholesterol levels. Although the exact mechanism for lowering cholesterol levels is not known, it is hypothesized that with increased blood flow there is increased fat burning and greater filtration through the liver, so much of the unhealthy cholesterol is eliminated over time.

LDL Cholesterol- AKA "Loser" Cholesterol
HDL Cholesterol – AKA "Helper" Cholesterol

Be patient when it comes to lowering your cholesterol levels. Compliance with current medications, a healthy diet, and a regular exercise regimen takes time to bring your levels back to normal.

Being informed about which kinds of cholesterols are healthy is another key for success. One of the easiest ways to start thinking about LDL and HDL cholesterol is by the first letter in the acronyms. You can associate LDL with "loser" and HDL with "helper."

LDL Cholesterol

Low-Density Lipoprotein (LDL) is known as the **bad** form of cholesterol. LDL cholesterol tends to stick to the sides of arteries and increase the possibility of heart disease, coronary artery disease, and other medical complications. Statin drugs prescribed by a doctor help control high cholesterol levels, but simply relying on the medications for a long-term change is unwise. Take the initiative to exercise regularly and eat fewer saturated fats and trans fats.

Foods High in LDL Cholesterol
Bacon
Butter
Cheese
Cheeseburgers
French Fries
Fried Foods
Margarine
Processed Foods
Red Meat

HDL Cholesterol

High-Density Lipoprotein (HDL) is known as **good** cholesterol, as it can transport LDL cholesterol away from the body. Higher levels of HDL cholesterol are known to **decrease** the risk of stroke, diabetes, and atherosclerosis. That's a great thing.

Foods High in HDL Cholesterol
Beans
Fish
Fruits
Legumes
Olive oil
Whole Wheat Breads

Triglycerides

Triglycerides represent the majority of fat in your blood and are determined by the cumulative amount of saturated, unsaturated, and polyunsaturated fats present in your body. The lower the number, the healthier your blood profile. This number is primarily based off of your current level of health, primary fat storage locations, overall diet, and exercise patterns. Think of triglycerides as an "overall picture" of your blood health.

It is very important to have your triglycerides under control. Excessive stores of triglycerides can increase the risk of atherosclerosis (hardening and narrowing of the arteries) and heart disease. Eating a healthy diet can help balance your triglyceride levels as fewer unhealthy fats will be present.

Your LDL, HDL and Triglyceride levels are directly linked to how healthy your heart and arteries are. The more LDL fat you intake, the higher risk of heart disease, stroke and atherosclerosis are.

A poor diet with poor lifestyle habits is often a primary indicator for elevated triglyceride levels. Lifestyle habits such as smoking, poorly controlled diabetes, excessive alcohol consumption, and being overweight/obese are a few avenues that inadvertently increase triglyceride levels.

Blood Results and Your Levels

LDL, HDL, and triglyceride levels are important to consider when looking at *any* diet. Total cholesterol levels can be determined by a doctor with a blood test. If you have had blood tests and have your numbers, the chart below can give you a good idea of where you stand. If you have not had your blood taken recently, it would be a smart idea to have it done—most of the time only a finger prick is necessary.

LDL Cholesterol (Bad)

Optimal	<100
Near Optimal	100-129
Borderline High	130-159
High	160-189
Very High	190 and Above

HDL Cholesterol (Good)

High (Higher is Better)	60 or Above
Low	Below 40

Triglycerides

Normal	Below 150
Borderline High	150-199
High	200-499
Very High	500 or Above

Total Cholesterol

Desirable	Below 200
Borderline High	200-239
High	240 and Above

Bursting with Energy: What You Need to Know About Carbohydrates

What kind of relationship is worth having if there is no spontaneity, energy, or excitement? This is where carbohydrates come into play with the food relationship, as they like to keep things exciting.

Carbohydrates, a.k.a. "carbs," are the most important form of energy possible to the human body. Not only is the brain dependent upon carbs, but so is nearly every cell in your body. To keep things simple when we think about carbs, a few major key terms should come to mind: **simple carbs, complex carbs, starch, and fiber**. Each play a different role in the body, and they should therefore be considered important and included every day in your diet.

Any diet that tells you to eliminate carbohydrates is a diet that you want to stay away from. Carbohydrates should make up at least 30-60% of one's daily diet.

Let's go back to chemistry class. Remember all those weird drawings that looked like chains and maps, detailing how something is structured? These are known as an element's chemical structure. That's exactly how we need to think about simple and complex carbohydrates. Simple carbs and complex carbs are structured exactly as their names suggest.

The easiest way to think about this is that simple carbs comprise of a single or double chain link, while complex carbs are made up of multiple chain links, all combined to one another.

A chain that has multiple strong links is not only stronger than a single link but can also perform more tasks—and more efficiently. Don't settle for the simple and unstable sugars; go with complex carbs.

While complex carbohydrates may have the edge on simple carbs, both are very important for our body to function properly, so how can we apply this to our foods and what we should eat?

Simple Carbohydrates

Simple carbs provide the body with quick energy. Due to their simple structure, the body utilizes and burns up that energy extremely quickly. They are also described by other names: fructose, glucose, galactose, maltose, sucrose, and lactose.

With such a quick rush of energy from simple sugars, the body's glucose (sugar) levels rise sharply.
Multiple sharp rises and falls in blood sugar over time will increases your risk of Type II Diabetes.

The most prevalent side effect of simple carbs is feeling instant energy followed by a crash. A good example of this is how you feel after drinking an energy drink or soda or after eating a piece of candy or dessert.

Simple Sugar Top Picks
Honey
Fruit
Milk
Brown Sugar
Chocolate (Cacao and Dark)

Another side effect of eating too many simple carbs is fat storage. Remember, **any extra energy the body does not readily use will become stored as fat**. With so many foods and drinks full of simple carbs, your body tends to store all the excess fat from these calorie bombs. Eliminating sugary drinks and desserts filled with simple carbs will slim that waistline faster than running ever will.

20 Common Examples of Simple Carbs

Brown Sugar

Cake

Candy

Cereal

Chocolate

Corn Syrup

Cream of Wheat / Grits

Dried Fruits

Flour

Fruit

Fruit Juice

Honey

Milk

Molasses

Pasta (white flour)

Pie

Soda

Table Sugar

Table Syrups

White Rice

Not all simple sugars are bad. The amount consumed in a single sitting or throughout the day is what makes simple sugars dangerous. Many simple sugars are so dense with calories that once we reach the point of satiety, we have already consumed more calories than our bodies need.

Many simple sugars are synonymous with preservatives, sweets, highly packaged foods, and long-term health issues. The top picks for simple sugars are ones that are less likely to be consumed in mass quantities. Bottom line: **be cautious when it comes to simple sugars**. Don't let them ruin all of your effort in a single meal.

When most people think about "sugar," they think cookies and candy. However, when talking about carbohydrates, they are simply a measurement for how complex the foods are.

Complex Carbohydrates

Complex carbohydrates also provide the body with energy like simple carbs, just at a slower rate. There is still a small spike in blood sugar levels, but they are broken down and utilized more efficiently over time. This is because of their complex chemical structure. The reduction in blood sugar spikes and increase in *sustained energy* makes complex carbohydrates the preferred choice. With energy being stored and utilized more efficiently, there is less chance of fat storage.

When it comes down to choosing between simple and complex

Choosing complex carbs to eat instead of simple carbs will keep you fuller for longer and reduce your risk of developing Type II Diabetes.

carbohydrates, **complex carbs should be your first choice**. Not only are they better for your health but are also typically less processed or manufactured.

Complex Carbohydrates Top Picks
Barley
Beans
Black Beans
Brown Rice or Wild Rice
Couscous
Greek and Low Fat Yogurt
Lentils and Legumes
Nuts
Oat Bran
Potatoes
Pumpkin and Squash
Quinoa
Seeds
Soymilk
Steel Grain Oatmeal
Sweet Potatoes (Yams)
Vegetables
Wheat Germ
Whole Wheat Bread & Tortillas
Whole Wheat Pasta

Low and No Carbohydrate diets are difficult to adhere to long-term. Although results of quick loss will be evident, a well-rounded diet with exercise is the safest and most sustainable method for weight loss.

Starch

Starches are complex carbohydrates. They are more advanced complex carbohydrates, as their chemical structure is made up of hundreds to thousands of sugars linked together. This makes them take the longest amount of time to breakdown out of all conventional complex carbs. Starches are only broken down by the body's digestion process. This is one reason why foods like potatoes and cereals become sweeter in your mouth the longer you chew, because your saliva is already beginning to break down the structure and release the sugars.

Starches are an important aspect of any healthy diet. Many starchy foods are full of vitamins and minerals; however, as healthy as

Most Americans are deficient in starch and fiber, both of which are key components of a healthy diet. Increasing your intake of whole wheat breads, fruits, and vegetables will help to reduce potential health problems and diseases in the future.

they are, they are also packed full of energy (sugar). This means starches should be proportioned appropriately and not overeaten. **Overconsumption is the main problem when eating starches or complex carbs.** It's not that they are bad, but because we tend to eat so many of them in such a short span of time, the body begins to store the excess energy as fat.

Diets that focus on limiting or eliminating carbohydrates have gained fame due to supposed drastic amounts of weight loss. However, once carbs are reintroduced, weight often rebounds back to pre-diet numbers.

20 Common Starches

Asparagus

Barley

Beans

Bread

Cereal

Corn

Lentils

Onions

Pasta

Pastries

Plantain

Potatoes

Quinoa

Rice

Seeds

Sorghum

Squash

Tortillas

Wheat

Yams

The Carbohydrate Catchall: The Glycemic Index

Maintaining safe blood sugar levels is something to consider when thinking long-term with your food relationship. Not all carbohydrates raise your blood sugar the same, so it is important to differentiate between each of them. Fortunately for you, the Glycemic Index is the tool that divides foods based upon their sugar content.

The Glycemic Index is broken down into three different groups: high, medium, and low. The number 100 in this index is the highest number, indicating the greatest sugar spike possible within the body. The higher the glycemic number, the greater the chance of fat storage and increased hunger. The glycemic index further reinforces the need to eat healthy and wholesome food. Do your best to stick to the medium and low categories. While this is an abridged list, it will help you know which foods are more beneficial than others.

The Glycemic Index

High (85-100)	Medium (60-85)	Low (<60)
Syrup	Banana	Apple
Crackers	Oatmeal	Beans
Soda	Whole Grain Breads	Milk
White Bread	Yams	Yogurt
Raisins	Corn	Lentils
Molasses	Potato Chips	Chick Peas

Fiber: Keeping Things Smooth

Even though fiber is one of the least considered aspects of a healthy food relationship, it is necessary for everything to run smoothly through your body. Fiber, a.k.a. roughage, primarily makes up of the structural components of plants and helps the movement of food material through the bowels. Fiber is also a type of carbohydrate. It is found solely in plant products, as meat and animal products do not contain any fiber. The body is unable to digest fiber or use it for energy, but it is put to good use in the gastrointestinal tract.

To keep things operating effectively, fiber is extremely important to heart, blood, and colon health. It is recommended to consume about 28g of fiber a day for a 2,000-calorie diet. One medium sized apple contains about 3.7g of fiber.

There are two types of fiber: soluble fiber and insoluble fiber. Soluble is a term that simply means broken down or dissolved by water. Therefore, some fibers are broken down by water and some aren't. Both soluble and insoluble fiber are found in fruits, veggies, grains, and oats. The amount of fiber differs in every food and is never exactly the same.

Men need to eat more fiber than women. Men should ingest about 38g of fiber per day, whereas women typically only require 25g.
After the age of 50, the daily intake for men is reduced to 30g and to 21g for women.

Soluble fiber plays a big role in blood sugar absorption, improves the overall health of the colon, and lowers blood cholesterol levels. Insoluble fiber helps with digestion,

increasing the rate in which food can move through the colon—
helping to prevent colon cancer.

20 Common Sources of Fiber

Apples
Bananas
Black Beans
Blueberries
Broccoli
Brown Rice
Corn
Dry Roasted Almonds and Peanuts
Grapes
Green Peas
Kidney Beans
Oat Bran
Oatmeal
Oranges
Potatoes
Prunes
Spinach
Squash
White Beans
Whole-Wheat Bread

Lean Mean Love Machine:
What You Need to Know About Protein

**Protein is a food relationship must. Everything centers
around protein from portion sizes to daily percentages.**
Proteins act as building blocks for your body's cells, help with
muscle contraction, and aid the immune system, as well as many

other essential life functions. Proteins are also responsible for the development of muscles, skin, bones, organs, and nearly everything else in the body.

Top Meat Proteins Ranked From Best to Worst
Fish
Chicken
Lean Game Meat
(Venison)
Turkey
Beef
Pork
Shrimp / Shellfish
Top Non-Meat Proteins
Soy beans / Soy Nuts
Eggs
Almonds / Various Nuts
Lentils / Beans
Peanut Butter
Plain Greek Yogurt
Tofu / Tempeh / Seitan
Milk
Spinach
Kale
Broccoli
Green Beans
Quinoa
Edamame
Chia Seeds

With all the responsibilities of protein in the body, it is important to try eating a protein at every meal. Proteins taste great and increase satiety, while providing our bodies with essential vitamins and nutrients. Proteins are typically associated with meat (most protein per gram) but are also abundant in many plant sources like beans and legumes. Therefore, there is no excuse not to eat proteins, as they accommodate every single diet.

Because proteins contain only 4 calories per gram, they provide fewer calories than fat per gram, which will help you eat fewer calories throughout the day. Protein also takes longer to burn, as it is not used as a primary energy source for the body. Centering your meals on proteins will keep you fuller for longer and accumulate fewer overall calories throughout the day.

Don't forget when choosing proteins to **go with lean proteins.** Typically, animal meats contain fat that surrounds the muscle tissue, and the fat is not beneficial for hypertension or hyperlipidemia (high blood pressure and high cholesterol). Consider this over-simplified explanation: the more fat, the less meat. Meat proteins are unique, containing more protein per serving than plants and vegetables. Consuming your protein through plant sources is a very healthy method of eating your protein, but keep in mind that you typically need to eat much more to get the same amount of protein.

How much protein should I eat each per day?

It is recommended to consume about 0.8g/kg of protein daily if you are not physically active. This is simply to properly maintain body functions, etc. If you are exercising or weightlifting, it is often recommended to consume 1.5g-2.0g/kg per day of protein. Keep in mind that protein's function is cell growth and structure, not energy production. Because exercise breaks down the muscle, protein helps not only to build it back but also build it back stronger than before.

Instead of breaking protein consumption down by grams or kilograms, you can break

Increasing your protein intake beyond the maintenance stage should be combined with increased water intake as well as a regular exercise regimen (3+ days a week). Always see your doctor before starting any exercise regimen.

it down into percentages. Although every diet is different and a dietician/ nutritionist is the best option for critiquing your daily intake percentages, the average person should try to consume anywhere from 10-35% of protein per day. The more exercise, the more protein you will likely need to consume.

If you are looking to get a little bit more advanced than simple percentages, here are some protein consumption guidelines. Based on a 2,000-calorie/day diet, it is recommended to have around 10-35% protein intake or about 200-700 calories worth.

Based on your current weight (1 kg = 2.2lbs)
Weights are rounded for simplification

100 lbs. = 46 kg	125 lbs. = 57 kg	150 lbs. = 68 kg	175 lbs. = 80 kg
200 lbs. = 91 kg	225 lbs. = 102 kg	250 lbs. = 114 kg	275 lbs. = 125 kg
300 lbs. = 136 kg	325 lbs. = 148 kg	350 lbs. = 159 kg	375 lbs. = 170 kg

Recommendations for protein intake, per day

Maintenance	0.8-1.1g per kg or 0.5 per lb.
Muscle Mass	1.2-1.7g per kg or 0.5-0.8g per lb.
Major Mass	1.8-2.0g per kg or 1.5g per lb.

Getting Buzzed?
What You Need to Know About Alcohol

Alcohol is neither categorized as a macronutrient or micronutrient. While alcohol does contain relatively high amounts of calories per gram (7 kcal/g), it is caloric dense with little to no nutritional benefit of any kind. **Sugar and carbohydrates are the sources of calories with any alcoholic beverage.** Due to alcohol's lack of nutrition, it is only recommended to have one drink for women and two drinks for men per day.

As much fun as a buzz can be, excess consumption of alcohol can lead to the following physical and mental health problems:

> **Short-Term**: Impaired judgment, impaired motor skills, increased possibility of violent behavior, alcohol poisoning, and miscarriage or stillbirth for pregnant women
> **Long-Term:** High blood pressure, liver disease, heart disease, stroke, digestive problems, and cancer of the breast, mouth, throat, esophagus, liver and colon. Learning and memory problems, alcohol dependence, lack of motivation, depression, and anxiety

So, think twice before opening that bottle. Ask yourself if you need those calories, let alone want burn them off. The long-term detriments of alcohol may not be worth the short-term benefits. If you can control your intake and are drinking for the right reasons, then enjoy a cold one, my friend.

Unnecessary Relationship Shortcuts: What You Need to Know About Supplements and Dietary Products

Let's be clear: Supplements and dietary products are *not* necessary in any capacity if you are able to eat a well-balanced diet. **They should *not* be considered as a *primary* component of your food relationship unless prescribed by a doctor.**

One of the reasons why supplement and dietary products are enticing is the appeal to get results without any major effort. You can't expect to have a fantastic relationship with your spouse if you don't spend any time or extra effort with them, so why should your food relationship be any different? If it sounds too good to be true, it probably is. The companies that manufacture these products are making big money on consumers that don't want to take the time to make their meals, workout long enough, or recover properly.

I'm not completely against supplements and some dietary products, but there needs to be in-depth research done on whatever product you are using prior to purchase. You will be amazed to discover how many fillers, preservatives, illegal substances, and unknown additives are incorporated in popular supplements. Research on a particular product should be performed utilizing non-affiliated sources. Non-affiliated sources will help confirm or deny the claims without coercion to purchase from a certain brand or company.

Supplement and dietary product companies are raking in billions of dollars each year, so you will be exposed to many ads and marketing campaigns nearly everywhere you go. Many people who get sucked into the pyramid schemes of weight loss can spend hundreds of dollars a month on shakes and powders. What if you spent that money on *real* food to put in your body rather than the overly processed powders, bars, and shakes? Your body would thank you.

The absolute best method to achieve results, hands down, is to put in time and effort—in the kitchen and at the gym. If you cut corners here or there, over time it will show. Let's be honest, no single "diet program" is sustainable year after year. The only long lasting diet is eating healthy and being diligent, day-in and day-out, growing a simple and healthy food relationship.

Amino Acids, commonly known as BCAA's (Branch Chain Amino Acids), are small building blocks that help make up proteins and other foods. They are commonly recommended by supplement shops to aid with recovery from strenuous exercise, and they are often synonymous with the bodybuilding community. Although the powdered supplements may be beneficial after rigorous training, you can obtain all of your essential amino acids through a well-balanced diet. Maintaining a well-balanced diet should be the priority over choosing a powdered and highly manufactured alternative. The Essential Amino Acids: Isoleucine, Leucine, Lysine, Methionine, Phenylalanine, Threonine, Tryptophan, Valine, and Histidine

Supplement Challenge Questions

If you are considering buying a supplement or dietary product, answer these following questions before you buy.

Why am I taking this product? Know the specific reason.

How much does this cost, and am I willing to pay for the product from here on out? Monthly cost?

What is even in this product? Look up EACH ingredient. If there are more than 10, you should consider looking elsewhere.

Does the FDA regulate this product?

Is this product for short-term or long-term use?

What are the side effects of this product? (Heart racing, upset stomach, irritability, sleeplessness, etc.)

Does my doctor or nutritionist recommend this product?

Does this product have any negative interactions with my medical history or other medications that I am taking? (Consult a doctor/ pharmacist / nutritionist)

Am I simply too lazy to eat better and workout, so I take this product instead?

Is this product or similar products on the High Risk List (U.S. Anti-Doping Agency)?

There is so much conflicting data on thousands of products, which is why it is imperative to simply eat simple, eat healthy, and exercise. **Don't be deceived by marketing gimmicks that make you feel inferior or feel like you need their products to succeed.**

Commonly Found Products

Beet Powder
Brain Health
Caffeine
Fast-Digesting Protein Powders
Inflammation and Immune System Boosters
Joint Health
Pre-Probiotics
Pre-Workout Powders
Slow Digestive Blends
Time Released Carbohydrate/Protein Blends
Vision Health
Vitamins

Leucine Rich Essential Amino Acids

Here is a list of some quality leucine rich essential amino acid foods/products that are worth looking into as they help stimulate Muscle Protein Synthesis (MPS). Simply put, diets with higher leucine rich foods combined with exercise will bolster the growth of muscle. **Notice that most are not supplements and can be incorporated into your regular diet.**

**Top Leucine Rich Essential
Amino Acids: Cheese
and Dairy Based**

Based on mg of Leucine
per oz (28,349 mg /oz)
Whey Protein Isolate –
2772 mg
Casein Hydrolysate –
2529 mg
Parmesan Cheese –
1124 mg
Dried Milk – 992 mg
Swiss Cheese – 829 mg
Fontina Cheese – 746 mg
Hard Goat Cheese –
737 mg
Edam or Gouda Cheese
718 mg
Cottage Cheese –
312 mg
Greek Yogurt – 177 mg
1% Milk – 108 mg

**Top Leucine Rich
Essential Amino Acids:
Plant Based**

Soy Protein Isolate –
2240 mg
Vital Wheat Gluten –
1904 mg
Seaweed Dried –
1385 mg
Soy Flour - 1072 mg
Cottonseed Meal –
939 mg
Raw Soybeans – 927 mg
Pumpkin/Squash Kernels
782 mg
Sunflower Kernels –
351 mg
Yellow Whole Grain
Cornmeal – 246 mg
Cooked Lentils – 183 mg
Regular Tofu – 172 mg
Oatmeal Bread – 164 mg

**Top Leucine Rich Essential Amino Acids:
Animal Based**
Egg White Solids –2464 mg
Dried Egg Whites –1875 mg
Whole Dried Eggs –1185 mg
Dried Egg Yolk –843 mg
Cooked Bacon –842 mg
Bison –811 mg
Lean Beef –804 mg
Veal / Lean Lamb Cuts – 774 mg
Chicken Breast –766 mg
Elk –741 mg
Lean Pork Cuts –725 mg
Moose –721 mg
Fresh Cooked Tuna – 681 mg
Lean Turkey / Ostrich –673 mg
Light Tuna / Salmon / Sword Fish- 580 mg
Hard Boiled Egg – 537 mg

Breaking Up with Gluten-Free

Before we address Gluten-Free diets, we should discuss
exactly what gluten is. The term "gluten" is a generalized name
for a group of proteins (primarily glutenin and gliadin) that are
commonly found in wheat products like wheat, rye, barley,
triticale, malt, regular oats, brewer's yeast, and wheat starch.
These proteins help foods maintain their shape and give dough its
elastic-like properties.

In recent years, gluten-free diets and gluten-free foods have exploded in popularity due to their endorsement by famous celebrities, various literature, and even some "nutrition" programs. These endorsements claim that weight loss, increased energy levels, and a better digestive system are all possible with a gluten-free diet. However, despite these claims, **gluten-free diets have not been proven to promote weight loss, increase energy, or relieve gastrointestinal issues.** The primary cause for weight loss and other associated symptoms is simply from making conscious decisions about what foods they eat. This is similar to any other diet on the market.

Oddly enough, gluten-free products often contain *more* preservatives and artificial flavors than regular food. This is to increase flavor and shelf life of the products. Gluten-free products contain fewer vitamins, cause decreases in beneficial gut bacteria, are more expensive, and contain little or no fiber. Just because there is an endorsement by a celebrity or your friend touts the "results" does not mean the claims are legitimate.

What about those who really need to eat gluten-free diets? Those who need to eat a gluten-free diet are a very small portion of our population. This small segment (1% of the *entire* population) has a gluten intolerance or gluten sensitivity. The two primary diagnoses are that of Celiac Disease (CD) and Non-Celiac Gluten Sensitivity (NCGS). Each diagnosis deals primarily with symptoms like stomach pain, diarrhea, and bloating. If for some reason you think you may have CD or NCGS, have it diagnosed by a doctor. They can perform a blood test and/or small intestine biopsy to see if you have gluten sensitivity. This is the only way to *truly* determine if you should go gluten-free.

Overall, with an extremely low diagnosis of CD and NCGS (86% of the complaints about gluten-related issues in their diets were only *self-perceived*, backed with absolutely no diagnosis of any kind), it is best to stay away from gluten-free diets. These diets are not beneficial for your body or your food relationship. Save your money and eat the real thing.

Nutritional Science Summary

This nutritional science section is just a small blip on the radar in comparison to all of the fantastic food science literature out there. Although concise in its nature, this section should help you dissect your food relationship a little deeper than before. With a basic understanding of what certain foods contain and why, you can now make more educated decisions next time you go shopping or visit your favorite restaurant.

Knowing about healthier foods won't do anything though until you actually eat them on a regular basis. Developing the habit to eat food that is good does take time, but most of the effort can be mitigated through proper tracking of your macronutrients (Carbs, Fats, Proteins) and micronutrients (Vitamins, Minerals).

It cannot be stressed enough that eating less processed foods is significantly better for your body. Throughout this section, it's been shown that processed foods and fatty meats will take a toll on your body in the long run. Although our bodies are efficient machines and can deal with almost anything, putting in the wrong fuel year-after-year is proven to lead to many comorbidities and even early death.

Next time you are tempted to eat unhealthy foods, just think about what those foods are doing to the inside of your body.

Sleeping on the Couch: Bad Food Decisions

No decision in a relationship comes without consequences, good or bad. It is easy to make poor decisions when we are rushed for time, tired, or hungry. Anytime our bodies are in need of an extra boost of energy, we eat whatever is close to use, often regretting it later.

This section was created so you can actually see just how much unhealthy food is out there and how much exercise is needed to simply burn it off. Marketing campaigns, slick slogans, and BOGO deals may sound appealing, but they are probably the last things your body needs. After all, it is easier to eat the terrible foods than to burn them off. Don't commit a nutritional crime and make your body pay the penalty.

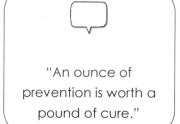

"An ounce of prevention is worth a pound of cure."

Eating poorly works similar to having a criminal record. The more crimes you commit, the harder it is to get clean and get out of jail. If you want to indulge in poor eating habits, don't be surprised if you see the weight stack on after a couple weeks. Don't forget that food crimes committed year after year can do permanent damage to your body in the form of heart disease, Type II Diabetes, high cholesterol, and high blood pressure.

The penalty is based off of jogging one mile, average speed. Jogging one mile burns approximately 120 calories. Burning off 600 calories takes about on average one hour on of brisk jogging at 5 mph.

Liquid Calories

The Crime	Calories	Sugar (g)	Fat (g)	Carbs (g)	Salt (mg)	The Penalty: Miles
Burger King Oreo Milk Shake (Large)	730	121	19	100	550	6.08
Coca Cola (20 oz)	240	65	0	65	75	2
Gatorade (591 ml)	150	35	0	38	250	1.25
Gold Peak Sweet Tea (18.5 oz)	190	48	0	48	50	1.58
Mountain Dew (20 oz)	290	77	0	77	105	2.4
Pepsi (20 oz)	250	69	0	69	55	2.08
Red Bull (12 oz)	168	37	0.3	40	140	1.4
Rock Star (16 oz)	200	54	0	54	38	1.6
Sonic's Peanut Butter Fudge Shake (Large)	1940	165	122	193	1080	16.1
Starbucks Iced Peppermint White Chocolate Mocha (Venti)	710	108	24	112	270	5.9

Alcoholic Liquid Calories

The Crime	Calories	The Penalty: Miles
Bud Light Lime-a-Rita (8 oz)	220	1.8
Everclear (1.5 oz)	226	1.8
Long Island Ice Tea (12 oz)	529	4.4
Margarita (12 oz)	417	3.4
Pina Colada (12 oz)	366	3
Samuel Adams Double Bock (12 oz)	230	1.9
Vodka and Red Bull (12 oz)	366	3

Candy and Sweets Calories

The Crime	Calories	Sugar (g)	Fat (g)	Carbs (g)	Salt (mg)	The Penalty: Miles
Breyers Cookies n' Cream Ice Cream (1/2 Cup)	140	15	4.5	23	80	1.16
Cotton Candy Express (2 oz)	210	-	0	52.5	-	1.75
M&M's (1.5 oz)	220	21	11	25	20	1.8
Hershey Kiss (9 pieces)	230	21	13	24	35	1.9
Kit Kat (1 bar or 1.5 oz)	218	20	11	27	23	1.8
Pop Tarts (2 Pastries)	400	32	10	76	340	3.3
Reese's Butter Cup (1 cup)	87	8	5	9	61	0.7
Snickers	215	20	11	28	83	1.8

Food Calories

The Crime	Calories	Sugar (g)	Fat (g)	Carbs (g)	Salt (mg)	The Penalty: Miles
Banquet Salisbury Steak Meal	350	11	14	44	1,340	2.9
Burger King Double Whopper	830	13	50	57	1,040	6.9
Taco Bell Volcano Nachos	990	7	59	94	1840	8.25
McDonald's Big Mac	550	9	29	46	970	4.58
McDonald's Big Breakfast with Hotcakes (Regular Size)	1090	17	56	111	2150	9.08
Oscar Mayer Beef Hotdogs (1 Link)	130	1	12	0	330	1.1
Stouffer's Fettuccini Alfredo (1 Container)	570	5	27	55	850	4.75
Kraft Easy Mac (1 Container)	450	10	9	26	920	3.75
Wendy's Baconator	940	9	56	41	1,890	7.8
Hot Pockets Pepperoni Pizza (2 Pack)	640	3	15	35	700	5.3

Tying the Knot

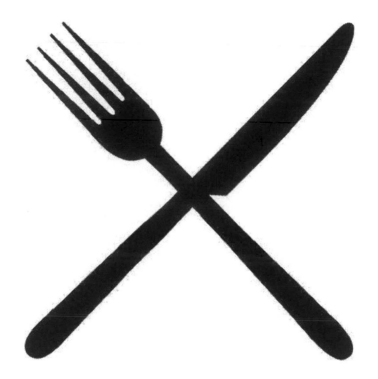

Love Should Be Like Fine Wine: It Gets Better with Time

The journey to eating healthier starts with you and ends with you. **You are the primary determining factor for your success.** The more time you spend working towards a healthier lifestyle, the quicker you will get results. This is why it is crucial to keep tangible short-term and long-term goals in mind every day that you wake up. Without attainable goals, we set ourselves up for failure. This is the opposite of what anyone wants and the exact opposite of what your body needs. You owe it to yourself and your loved ones to take care of yourself. We only live this one life, so let's make the most out of it.

Here are some questions to review. Over time, some of these answers will change, and that's okay. Revisit the sections as needed to continue strengthening your nutritional journey day-in and day-out.

What are your intrinsic motivations for eating healthier? Have these motivations changed at all throughout this book? If so, how?

What dietary goals do you have? Weight loss, maintenance, or weight gain?

What are you going to do differently both with your diet and lifestyle habits?

Name at least five foods that you removed from your kitchen / pantry and their healthier replacements.

How many people are you typically shopping for?

What are going to be your three primary sources of protein in your diet?

What is your daily caloric intake?

How many calories make up a pound of fat?

How many calories are present in one gram of protein, carbohydrate, fat, and alcohol?

How many ounces of water are you supposed to drink each day?

What are your biggest temptations when it comes to eating outside of your home?

Name three foods that are your vices? Name three healthy substitutes for each vice.

List seven vegetables that you enjoy eating.

Name three healthy choices for breakfast.

What are two types of bread recommended to purchase?

Which type of fat is the least healthy and should be avoided?

How many days a week do you exercise?

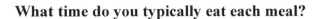

What time do you typically eat each meal?

What long-term health goals do you have for yourself?

What are you doing to achieve these goals, every day?

Keeping your internal motivation(s) in the forefront of your mind will lend to greater success and fulfillment throughout the upcoming days. This is especially true when confronted with bouts of laziness, fatigue, or busy schedules. The relationship you forge with food is something that no diet or quick weight loss program can develop. If you choose to start a better relationship with food, it will have its ups and downs like any other relationship. However, there will be more ups than downs, and your knowledge of food will only grow and strengthen as time passes. You will soon be able to see through the gimmicks and navigate the aisles of a store without second thought. When presented with temptations of unhealthy foods that could sabotage your goals, you will be able to navigate them appropriately with the knowledge gained from this book.

I have faith in you that with the proper motivating factors, support from your loved ones, perseverance, and diligence, **you will be able to accomplish any nutritional goal you set**. Creating a simple and healthy food relationship will be the best decision that could ever make for your body!

Citations

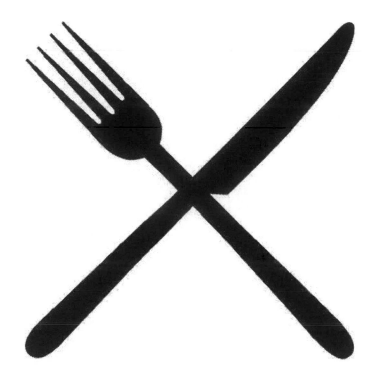

Citations

1 oz Boneless Beefsteak. Fatsecret.
https://www.fatsecret.com/calories-nutrition/generic/beef-steak-ns-as-to-fat-eaten?portionid=1935&portionamount=1.000 : . July, 2016.

Alcohol Calorie Calculator. Rethinking Drinking – Alcohol & Your Health.
https://www.rethinkingdrinking.niaaa.nih.gov/tools/Calculators/calorie-calculator.aspx : . December, 2016.

Alcohol and Public Health. Frequently Asked Questions. Center for Disease Control and Prevention Website.
http://www.cdc.gov/alcohol/faqs.htm : . October, 2016. December, 2016.

Andrei, Mihai. Is Organic Food Actually Better? Here's what the science says. ZME Science.
http://www.zmescience.com/other/science-abc/organic-food-science02092015/ : . September, 2015. August, 2016.

Appendix 9. Alcohol. The Office Of Disease Prevention and Health Promotion.
https://health.gov/dietaryguidelines/2015/guidelines/appendix-9/ : December, 2016.

Baechle TR, Earle RW. Essentials of Strength Training and Conditioning. 3rd ed. Leeds: Human Kinetics; 2008.

Barclay, Laurie. Liver Detoxification – Fact or Fad? WebMD Website. http://www.webmd.com/men/features/liver-detoxification----fact-fad#1 : . December, 2001. November, 2016.

Britten, Patricia. Marcoe, Kristin. Yamini, Sedigheh. Davis, Carole. Development of Food Intake Patterns for the MyPyramid Food Guidance System. United States Department of Agriculture.
https://www.cnpp.usda.gov/sites/default/files/myplate_miplato/JNEBDevelPatterns.pdf : . November / December 2006. December, 2016.

Burger King Nutrition Facts & Calorie Information A Nutrition Guide to the Burger King Menu for Healthy Eating. Nutrition-Charts Website. http://www.nutrition-charts.com/burger-king-nutritional-information/ : . November, 2016.

Capannolo, A. Viscido, A. Barkad, M.A. Valerii, G. Ciccone, F. Melideo, D. Frieri, G. Latella G. Non-Celiac Gluten Sensitivity among Patients Perceiving Gluten-Related Symptoms. Karger Medical and Scientific Publishers Website. http://www.karger.com/Article/Abstract/430090 : . August, 2015. December, 2016.

Cataldo, Donna. Blair, Matthew. PROTEIN INTAKE FOR OPTIMAL MUSCLE MAINTENANCE, *ACSM's Consumer Information Committee*. 2015. Page 1.

Cattlemen's Beef Board And National Cattlemen's Beef Association. Many of America's Favorite Cuts Are Lean. Nutrition.org. http://www.beefitswhatsfordinner.com/CMDocs/BIWFD/FactSheets/Many_Of_Americas_Favorite_Cuts_Are_Lean.pdf : . July, 2016.

Cholesterol Levels: What You Need to Know. NIH MedicinePlus Website. https://medlineplus.gov/magazine/issues/summer12/articles/summer12pg6-7.html : . Summer, 2012. November, 2016.

Collins, Sonya. Alkaline Diets. WebMD Website. http://www.webmd.com/diet/a-z/alkaline-diets : . March, 2016. November, 2016.

Cooper, Jamie. Ellis, Dave. Nutritional Myths and Practices of the Elite Athlete Implications for Active, Non. YouTube Website. https://www.youtube.com/watch?v=elaWrhSJ4Og&t=19s&index=6&list=PLH3yLqj49r0_g-rlWCKwtm4T6OUcr-aAj : . November, 2016. November, 2016.

DASH Diet. A World Report U.S. News. http://health.usnews.com/best-diet/dash-diet : . November, 2016.

Dictionary. Merriam Webster. https://www.merriam-webster.com/dictionary/motivation: . December, 2016.

Do You Know How Food Portions Have Changed In 20 Years? National Heart, Lung, and Blood Institute. http://www.nhlbi.nih.gov/health/educational/wecan/portion/documents/PD1.pdf : . August, 2016.

Edgar, Julie. Types of Teas and Their Health Benefits. WebMD Website. http://www.webmd.com/diet/features/tea-types-and-their-health-benefits#1 : . March, 2009. August, 2016.

Ehrman JK, deJong A. ACSM's resource manual for Guidelines for exercise testing and prescription. Philadelphia: Wolters Kluwer Heslth/Lippincott Williams & Wilkins; 2010.

Fact Sheets - Alcohol Use and Your Health. Center for Disease Control and Prevention Website. http://www.cdc.gov/alcohol/fact-sheets/alcohol-use.htm : . July, 2016. December, 2016.

Fantar, Suzanne. Are Starches a Complex Carbohydrates? SFGate Website. http://healthyeating.sfgate.com/starches-complex-carbohydrate-7780.html : . November, 2016.

Fresh Pork From Farm To Table. United States Department of Agriculture. http://www.fsis.usda.gov/wps/portal/fsis/topics/food-safety-education/get-answers/food-safety-fact-sheets/meat-preparation/fresh-pork-from-farm-to-table/CT_Index : . July, 2016.

Fish and Omega-3 Fatty Acids. American Heart Association. http://www.heart.org/HEARTORG/HealthyLiving/HealthyEating/HealthyDietGoals/Fish-and-Omega-3-Fatty-Acids_UCM_303248_Article.jsp#.V_F8h5MrKu4 : . October, 2016. October, 2016.

Food and Nutrition Board, Institute of Medicine, National Academies. Dietary Reference Intakes (DRIs): Recommended Dietary Allowances and Adequate Intakes, Vitamins. https://www.nal.usda.gov/sites/default/files/fnic_uploads//RDA_AI_vitamins_elements.pdf : . August, 2016.

Fry, Fred. BBB – Various Shellfish-Associated Toxins. U.S. Department of Health and Human Services. http://www.fda.gov/Food/FoodborneIllnessContaminants/CausesOfIllnessBadBugBook/ucm070795.htm : . October, 2010. August, 2016.

Get Drunk Not Fat. http://getdrunknotfat.com/ : . December, 2016.

Getting your vitamins and minerals through diet. Harvard Medical School Website. http://www.health.harvard.edu/womens-health/getting-your-vitamins-and-minerals-through-diet : . July, 2009. August, 2016.

Gold Peak Sweet Tea. Gold Peak Tea & Coffee Website. http://www.goldpeakbeverages.com/gold-peak-products/tea/bottled/gold-peak-sweet-tea : . November, 2016.

Hall, Kate. Yes, GMOs Are Safe (Another Major Study Confirms. Forbes. http://www.forbes.com/sites/gmoanswers/2016/05/20/gmos-are-safe/#2afdb3d7119d : . May, 2016. August, 2016.

Harvard Women's Health Watch. The dubious practice of detox. Harvard Medical School Website. http://www.health.harvard.edu/staying-healthy/the-dubious-practice-of-detox : . May, 2008. November, 2016.

Health Benefits of Fish. Washington State Department of Health. http://www.doh.wa.gov/CommunityandEnvironment/Food/Fish/HealthBenefits : . July, 2016.

Healthy Weight. Harvard T.H. Chan School of Public Health. https://www.hsph.harvard.edu/nutritionsource/healthy-weight/ : . January 2017.

Healthwise, Incorporated. Vitamins: Their Functions and Sources - Topic Overview. WebMD Website. http://www.webmd.com/vitamins-and-supplements/tc/vitamins-their-functions-and-sources-topic-overview : . August, 2016.

Heller, Maria. What Is the DASH Diet? The Dash Diet Eating Plan. http://dashdiet.org/what_is_the_dash_diet.asp : . November, 2016.

Hitti, Miranda. Canned Fruits, Veggies Healthy, Too. WebMD Website. http://www.webmd.com/food-recipes/news/20070316/canned-fruits-veggies-healthy-too#1 : . March, 2007. August, 2016.

Johnson, Paul M. Kenny, Paul J. Dopamine D2 receptors in addiction-like reward dysfunction and compulsive eating in obese rats. Nature Neuroscience. Nature.com Website. http://www.nature.com/neuro/journal/v13/n5/abs/nn.2519.html : . March, 2010. December, 2016.

Kirkpatrick, Kristin. The Healthiest Breads: 6 Types Explained. The Huffington Post. http://www.huffingtonpost.com/2011/11/06/healthiest-breads_n_1078520.html : . May, 2016. August, 2016.

Kresser, Chris. Red Meat: It Does a Body Good! https://chriskresser.com/red-meat-it-does-a-body-good/ : . March, 2013. July, 2016.

Lee, Elizabeth. The Truth About Red Meat. WebMD Website. http://www.webmd.com/food-recipes/features/the-truth-about-red-meat#2 : . August, 2011. July, 2016.

Leech, Joe. The Alkaline Diet: An Evidence-Based Review. Authority Nutrition Website. https://authoritynutrition.com/the-alkaline-diet-myth/ : . November, 2016.

MacDonald, Ann. Why eating slowly may help you feel full faster. Harvard Medical School Website. http://www.health.harvard.edu/blog/why-eating-slowly-may-help-you-feel-full-faster-20101019605 : . October, 2010. December, 2016.

Magee, Elaine. Frozen Vegetables Are Hot!. WebMD Website. http://www.webmd.com/food-recipes/features/frozen-vegetables-are-hot#1 : . August, 2016.

Magee, Elaine. The Best Bread: Tips For Buying Breads. WebMD Website. http://www.webmd.com/food-recipes/features/the_best_bread_tips_for_buying_breads#1 : . 2009. August, 2016.

Martin, Laura J. Guide to a Healthy Kitchen – Tips for Reaping the Benefits of Whole Grains. WebMD. http://www.webmd.com/diet/healthy-kitchen-11/reaping-benefits-whole-grains : . May, 2016. August, 2016.

Mayo Clinic Staff. Mediterranean diet: A heart-healthy eating plan. Mayo Clinic Website. http://www.mayoclinic.org/healthy-lifestyle/nutrition-and-healthy-eating/in-depth/mediterranean-diet/art-20047801 : . May, 2016. November, 2016.

Mediterranean Diet. American Heart Association Website. http://www.heart.org/HEARTORG/HealthyLiving/HealthyEating/Mediterranean-Diet_UCM_306004_Article.jsp#.WDoJkKlrJmA : . October, 2016. November, 2016.

Nieman, David. Exercise Testing and Prescription, A Health-Related Approach, 7th Edition. New York, New York. McGraw-Hill; 2011. Page 223.

Nieman, David. Exercise Testing and Prescription, A Health-Related Approach, 7th Edition. New York, New York. McGraw-Hill; 2011. Pages 224-225.

Nieman, David. Exercise Testing and Prescription, A Health-Related Approach, 7th Edition. New York, New York. McGraw-Hill; 2011. Pages 223, 228, 230, 242.

Nieman, David. Exercise Testing and Prescription, A Health-Related Approach, 7th Edition. New York, New York. McGraw-Hill; 2011. Pages 231-232.

Nieman, David. Exercise Testing and Prescription, A Health-
    Related Approach, 7th Edition. New York, New York.
    McGraw-Hill; 2011. Page 266.

Nordqvist, Christian. Dietary Fiber: Why Do We Need It? Medical
    News Today Website.
    http://www.medicalnewstoday.com/articles/146935.php : .
    December, 2016. December, 2016.

Nordqvist, Christopher. What Are Calories? How Many Do We
    Need? Medical News Today Website.
    http://www.medicalnewstoday.com/articles/263028.php : .
    February, 2016. August, 2016.

Nordqvist, Joseph. Coffee: Health Benefits, Nutritional
    Informaton. Medical News Today.
    http://www.medicalnewstoday.com/articles/270202.php : .
    April, 2016. August, 2016.

Nutrient Data Laboratory. United States Department of
    Agriculture.
    http://www.ars.usda.gov/main/site_main.htm?modecode=
    80-40-05-25 : . August, 2016.

Nutrition-Healthy Living. American Heart Association.
    http://www.heart.org/HEARTORG/HealthyLiving/HealthyEati
    ng/Nutrition/Nutrition_UCM_310436_SubHomePage.jsp : .
    August, 2016.

Ohikuare, Judith. The 10 Highest & Lowest Calorie Drinks to
    Watch Out for Over Spring Break. HerCampus Website.
    http://www.hercampus.com/health/food/10-highest-
    lowest-calorie-drinks-watch-out-over-spring-break : . March,
    2014. November, 2016.

Peng, Tina. The Six Most Fattening Summer Cocktails. Newsweek
    Website. http://www.newsweek.com/six-most-fattening-
    summer-cocktails-90881 : . June, 2008. November, 2016.

Pepperoni Pizza. Hotpockets & Sandwiches Website.
    https://www.hotpockets.com/products/pepperoni-pizza-
    garlic-buttery-seasoned-crust/11595 : . November, 2016.

Perrella K, Cerny FJ. Hot Topics In Nutrition And How To Advise
    Your Client. ACSM's Health & Fitness Journal. 2017;21:13–8.

Pick From A Rainbow Of Beautiful Fruits and Veggies. Everyday
    Health. http://www.everydayhealth.com/healthy-recipe-
    pictures/pick-from-a-rainbow-of-beautiful-fruits-and-
    veggies.aspx : . May, 2011. August, 2016.

Potatoes, bread, rice, pasta and other starchy carbohydrates. British Nutrition Foundation Website. https://www.nutrition.org.uk/healthyliving/healthyeating/starchyfoods.html : . November, 2016. November, 2016.

Puckette, Madeline. Common Types of Wine (the top varieties). Wine Folly. http://winefolly.com/review/common-types-of-wine/ : . May, 2015. December, 2016.

Rivas, Anthony. Let's Get Drunk! The Healthiest Ways To Drink Alcohol. Medical Daily Website. http://www.medicaldaily.com/lets-get-drunk-healthiest-ways-drink-alcohol-269583 : . February, 2014. December, 2016.

Ross, Ken. Wine Press: Which wine has the fewest calories?. Mass Live. http://www.masslive.com/drinks/2014/01/wine_press_which_wine_has_the.html : . January, 2014. December, 2016.

Safe Eat of Shellfish. Oregon Health Authority. https://public.health.oregon.gov/HealthyEnvironments/Recreation/Documents/Shellfish-safety.pdf : . August, 2016.

SALISBURY STEAK MEAL WITH MASHED POTATOES. Banquet Website. http://www.banquet.com/classic-dinners/salisbury-steak-meal-mashed-potatoes : November, 2016.

Saturated Fats. American Heart Association Website. http://www.heart.org/HEARTORG/HealthyLiving/HealthyEating/Nutrition/Saturated-Fats_UCM_301110_Article.jsp#.V6ZeXJMrJmA : . October, 2016. November, 2016.

Scott, Jennifer R.. Calorie Counts for Alcoholic Drinks. Verywell. https://www.caloriecount.com/calories-alcoholic-drinks-ic1401 : . December, 2016. December, 2016.

Sifferlin, Alexandra. Fresh vs. Canned: Can You Get Healthy Food from a Can? Time. http://healthland.time.com/2012/04/23/fresh-vs-canned-can-you-get-healthy-food-from-a-can/slide/tuna/ : . April, 2012. August, 2016.

Smith, Janelle. What is Gluten? Celiac Disease Foundation Website. https://celiac.org/live-gluten-free/glutenfreediet/what-is-gluten/ : . December, 2016.

Sonic Nutritional Information. Sonic Restaurant Website. https://www.sonicdrivein.com/static/pdf/41682-33_NAT_F16_BRO_FA_LR1.pdf : Fall, 2016. November, 2016.

Starbucks Expresso Beverages. Starbucks Website.
https://www.starbucks.com/menu/catalog/nutrition?food=
all#view_control=nutrition&drink=espresso&food=bakery&fo
od=petites&food=bistro-boxes&food=hot-
breakfast&food=sandwiches-panini-and-wraps&food=ice-
cream&food=yogurt-and-fruit : . November, 2016.

TDM. The Most and Least Fattening Cuts of Steak-. Leon's
Restaurant. http://www.leonsrestaurant.com/fattening-
cuts-steak : March, 2014. July, 2016.

Teahan M. NESTA Fitness Nutrition Coach Program [Internet].
Rancho Santa Margarita, CA: John Spencer Ellis Enterprises
Inc.; 2017. Available from: http://fnc.nestaonline.com/wp-
content/uploads/2017/03/Fitness-Nutrition-Coach-
Manual.pdf

Tipton KD. Wolfe RR. Exercise, protein metabolism, and muscle
growth. PubMed
Website. https://www.ncbi.nlm.nih.gov/pubmed/11255140
: . March, 2001. December, 2016.

Tomato Soup. Cambell's Soups Website.
https://www.campbells.com/campbell-
soup/condensed/tomato-soup/ : . November, 2016.

The benefits of eating fish. Environmental Defense Fund.
http://seafood.edf.org/benefits-eating-fish : . July, 2016.

The Best Sustainable Fish to Eat in the Summer. Center For Food
Safety. http://www.centerforfoodsafety.org/healthy-
home/3274/cfs-healthy-home/tips-for-a-healthy-
home/3275/the-best-sustainable-fish-to-eat-in-the-summer :
. August, 2016.

The Reality Behind Gluten-Free Diets. UW Health
Website. http://www.uwhealth.org/nutrition-diet/the-
reality-behind-gluten-free-diets/31084 : . February, 2011.
December, 2016.

Trans Fats. American Heart Association Website.
http://www.heart.org/HEARTORG/HealthyLiving/HealthyEati
ng/Nutrition/Trans-
Fats_UCM_301120_Article.jsp#.V6eQe5MrL-Y: . October,
2015. November, 2016.

Triple Chocolate Cake. McCormick Website.
http://www.mccormick.com/recipes/dessert/triple-
chocolate-cake : . November, 2016.

Trumbo, Paula R. Nutrition & Supplement Facts Label Proposed Rule. U.S. Food and Drug Administration. http://www.fda.gov/downloads/Food/NewsEvents/Worksh opsMeetingsConferences/UCM403514.pdf : . August, 2016.

Tukey Bacon: How Healthy Is It Really? Cleveland Clinic. https://health.clevelandclinic.org/2015/07/turkey-bacon-how-healthy-is-it-really/ : . September, 2016.

Types of Carbohydrates. American Diabetes Association. http://www.diabetes.org/food-and-fitness/food/what-can-i-eat/understanding-carbohydrates/types-of-carbohydrates.html?referrer=https://www.google.com/ : . March, 2015. November, 2016.

United States Department of Agriculture. SATURATED, UNSATURATED, AND TRANS FATS. Choosemyplate.gov Website. http://www.choosemyplate.gov/saturated-unsaturated-and-trans-fats : . October, 2016. November, 2016.

Volta, U1. Caio, G. Tovoli, F. De Giorgio, R. Non-celiac gluten sensitivity: questions still to be answered despite increasing awareness. PubMed Website. https://www.ncbi.nlm.nih.gov/pubmed/23934026 : . September, 2013. December, 2016.

Ware, Megan. Milk: Health Benefits and Nutritional Information. Medical News Today. http://www.medicalnewstoday.com/articles/273451.php : . March, 2016. September, 2016.

What's In Food. Commonly Asked Questions (FAQs). Nutrition.gov Website. https://www.nutrition.gov/whats-food/commonly-asked-questions-faqs January, 2017. August, 2016.

White, Dana Angelo. Shellfish:Good or Bad?. The Foot Network. http://blog.foodnetwork.com/healthyeats/2010/02/09/shell fish-good-or-bad/ : . February, 2010. August, 2016.

Why Is It Important? President's Council on Fitness, Sports and Nutrition. https://www.fitness.gov/eat-healthy/why-is-it-important/ : . August, 2016.

Why Is It Important to Eat Vegetables? USDA Choosemyplate.gov https://www.choosemyplate.gov/vegetables-nutrients-health : . August, 2016.

Wright, Brierley. 30 Unhealthy Restaurant Menu Words to Avoid. EatingWell Website. http://www.eatingwell.com/blogs/diet_blog/30_unhealthy_

restaurant_menu_words_to_avoid : . August, 2013.
November, 2016.

Your Source for Nutritional Food Data. Nutrition-Charts Website.
http://www.nutrition-charts.com/ : November, 2016.

Zaxby's Nutritional Information. Zaxby's Restaurant.
https://www.zaxbys.com/zaxbys-nutritional-information/ : .
December, 2016.

Zeratsky, Katherine. Do detox diets offer and health benefits?
Mayo Clinic Website. http://www.mayoclinic.org/healthy-
lifestyle/nutrition-and-healthy-eating/expert-answers/detox-
diets/faq-20058040 : . March, 2015. November, 2016.

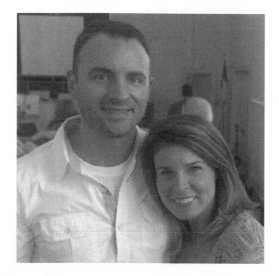

Brian Vernetti is an active American College of Sport Medicine (ACSM) Certified Personal Trainer, NESTA Fitness Nutrition Coach and USA Level 1 Weightlifting Coach, and career Firefighter and Emergency Medical Technician. He has a passion for all things fitness and health, and he strives to live his life in such a way that will inspire others to be the best version of themselves. His specialties are unique personal training programs, nutrition guidance/counseling, and interval training.

He is especially passionate about nutrition and recognizes the difficulties our society faces when beginning the journey to a healthy lifestyle. He wrote this book as a labor of love for all who have experienced nutrition confusion and repeated disappointment with fad diets and quick weight loss programs.

Brian currently resides with his wife in Baltimore, Maryland, and together they enjoy traveling and outdoor activities. He is also the owner and operator of Interval Athlete Fitness, a site dedicated to exercise, nutrition, and overall health: www.intervalathlete.com.

John 10:10

Made in the USA
Middletown, DE
06 February 2018